BETTER SEX THROUGH MINDFULNESS

Also Available from Lori A. Brotto:

*The Better Sex through Mindfulness Workbook:
A Guide to Cultivating Desire*

LORI A. BROTTO, PhD

Foreword by **EMILY NAGOSKI, PhD**

BETTER SEX THROUGH MINDFULNESS

How Women Can Cultivate Desire

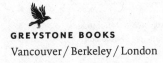

GREYSTONE BOOKS
Vancouver / Berkeley / London

Greystone Books Ltd.
greystonebooks.com

Cataloguing data available from Library and Archives Canada
ISBN 978-1-77164-235-4 (pbk.)
ISBN 978-1-77164-243-9 (epub)

Editing by Nancy Flight
Copyediting by Lesley Cameron
Cover and text design by Nayeli Jimenez
Printed and bound in Canada on FSC® certified paper by Friesens.
The FSC® label means that the materials used for the product have
been responsibly sourced.

Greystone Books thanks the Canada Council for the Arts, the British
Columbia Arts Council, the Province of British Columbia through
the Book Publishing Tax Credit, and the Government of Canada for
supporting our publishing activities.

Canada

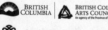
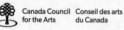
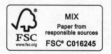

Greystone Books gratefully acknowledges the xʷməθkʷəy̓əm (Musqueam),
Sḵwx̱wú7mesh (Squamish), and səlilwətaɬ (Tsleil-Waututh) peoples on
whose land our Vancouver head office is located.

*To all the women who trusted that a fulfilling
sex life was a breath away.*

CONTENTS

FOREWORD

"**H**OORAY! AT LAST!"
That was my first thought when I got my hands on this important book.

My job is to travel around the world teaching women to embrace their sexuality with confidence and joy. It's the best job ever. And for more than a decade, I've been recommending mindfulness as a key to sexual well-being. Whether they're students, clients, readers, or strangers in airports who tell me about their sexual difficulties, whether they're distressed about sexual desire or arousal or orgasm or pain, and whether those difficulties seem to have appeared out of the blue or are tied to trauma or illness, the research is utterly convincing: mindfulness can help.

And if that student, client, or stranger wanted to know more about how to use mindfulness to improve her sex life, I'd tell her, "Read Lori Brotto's work. She's doing *amazing* research and clinical work on mindfulness and sexual well-being for women, including those recovering from sexual trauma or gynecological cancers."

The student or stranger would say, "That sounds perfect! What's her book called?"

Answer: "Well, she's written a lot of peer-reviewed academic journal articles…"

But now—Hooray! At last!—I can tell people, "It's called *Better Sex through Mindfulness*. It's simple, practical, science-based, and, above all, overflowing with *hope*."

Better Sex through Mindfulness delivers even more than the title promises. It provides historical context and scientific evidence that gently erase long-standing cultural myths about sex—like the idea that sexual desire should be automatic and that sexual activity should come naturally and easily. Or that sex has a role in reproduction but is a frivolous, self-indulgent activity when pursued for pleasure. Or that sexual desire diminishes as we age, no matter what. The book reassures us that women vary. We vary both from woman to woman and across our own individual lifespan. Brotto also demystifies the tremendously wide range of normal, healthy reasons why we might want, like, and decide to have sex: Sometimes for pleasure. Sometimes for procreation. Sometimes to make our partner happy. Sometimes just to help us fall asleep. And all of those reasons (and more!) are normal.

Above all, *Better Sex through Mindfulness* provides simple yet powerful exercises to help you, the reader, begin practicing mindfulness (or, if you already have a mindfulness practice, to deepen that practice) to expand your sexual well-being.

Our attention tends to be a little peripatetic even under the best of circumstances. As Brotto writes, "Our attention wanders like a puppy," and many of us have spent years training that puppy to wander in any direction except toward our internal sensations, especially our sexual sensations. As a result of negative sexual experiences and cultural messages, our attention has been trained to watch out for problems—to criticize our bodies, to monitor our responses during sex, and to worry about whether we're "doing it right" or even whether we should be doing it at all. Many of us have been taught, almost from the moment of our birth, to ignore or criticize or mistrust our sexual bodies.

Mindfulness is the practice of noticing what is happening inside us and of being kind to ourselves, even when we struggle to do so. Mindfulness means giving ourselves permission to pay attention—in a neutral, nonjudgmental way—to our bodies, our beliefs about sex, and our emotions related to sex. It means being patient and being kind to ourselves. And it means being nonjudgmental. That is the secret ingredient: nonjudgment. Mindfulness improves nonjudgmental attention, and nonjudgmental attention improves sexual well-being.

One of the beautiful aspects of mindfulness as a treatment for sexual difficulties is its gentleness. It isn't always necessary to dig into the details of past traumas or childhood adversity. With mindfulness, you can notice the residue of past painful experiences, and then you can release them. Instead of focusing on them, you notice them neutrally and allow them to move on.

At the heart of mindfulness lies a deep paradox: We facilitate change by *not trying to change.*

"Acceptance" is a difficult word to apply to sexual concerns. Women resist the idea, thinking, "If I accept my lack of desire, aren't I just accepting that I'll have to live with it forever?"

On the contrary, only by allowing ourselves to be fully aware of our internal experience can we understand it well enough to know what our bodies need.

For example, one evening in Portland, Oregon, after I had given a talk about the science of women's sexual well-being, a former student, whom I recognized and greeted with delight, came up to tell me her story.

She said, "The whole time I was in school, Emily, you kept saying, 'Mindfulness is good for you; you should try mindfulness. Mindfulness, mindfulness.' But every time I tried it, when my attention dropped down into my body, all I noticed were sirens and red flashing lights. And I thought, 'Why would I want to accept *that*? It's terrible!' But I kept trying, and I kept hearing sirens and seeing red flashing lights, until eventually I wondered if maybe that wasn't normal. So I went to the doctor, and it turns out I have fibromyalgia. I'd been living with pain every day and had not even known it wasn't normal. I had just blocked it from my attention so that I could cope."

My former student has continued practicing mindfulness as one of the evidence-based strategies that help her minimize the impact of her symptoms on her daily life. She finds the practice much easier now that she knows those sirens are nothing to be afraid of; they are a signal that her body is asking for help.

"And by the way," she said, "finally not being in pain all the time did fantastic things for my sex life."

If you allow your attention to drop down into your body and you find more suffering than you can tolerate, seek support from a professional, whether that's a therapist or a medical provider. Mindfulness is not only effective in repairing and expanding our sense of well-being (including our sexual well-being) but also in helping us hear our body's distress signals so that we can give it the support it needs and deserves.

But the first step is to turn toward our internal experience with nonjudgment. With acceptance.

At the end of the book, Brotto addresses those who feel they are "not wired for mindfulness." I appreciate that, because I am one of those people. The research convinces me that I should practice mindfulness, just as I should exercise and eat leafy

greens, so I do it—but boy, I am so bad at it. Even after meditating (badly) in some form or another for decades, I have yet to
experience more than fleeting moments, maybe a few minutes
at a time, of "mental stillness" or "inner peace."

But here is the astonishing truth that *Better Sex through Mindfulness* reveals: mindfulness is so powerful that it can work
even if you don't feel "wired" for it. If you're tuning in enough
to notice how noisy, cluttered, and wandering your mind is—if
you can notice that the puppy of your attention is just romp-
ing all over the place—you're doing it right. That's all it takes
for mindfulness to begin working its magic. All you have to
do is be kind to the puppy of your attention. Even when she
is wild and chaotic. Even—especially—when she is scared or
suffering. Mindfulness isn't about imposing stern discipline
on the puppy; it's about attending to her with patience and
nonjudgment, as you ask her to notice your internal sensations.

You are about to read a book full of wisdom, permission,
kindness, and hope. No matter who you are or what you're
experiencing with your sexuality, and no matter how "bad"
you believe you might be at mindfulness, the knowledge and
skills in this book can be transformative. Practice paying nonjudgmental attention to your internal sensations. It's even
simpler—and more powerful—than it sounds, and Dr. Lori
Brotto will show you the way.

EMILY NAGOSKI, PhD
New York Times bestselling author of *Come as You Are: The Surprising New Science That Will Transform Your Sex Life*

INTRODUCTION

ALTHOUGH PREVAILING SOCIETAL beliefs would suggest that sexual response is automatic, pleasurable, and universally desired, the reality is that female sexual dysfunction is extremely common around the world, with between 15 and 31 percent of women experiencing lasting and distressing sexual complaints. Female sexual dysfunction can affect one or more domains of sexuality (sexual desire, arousal, orgasm, and sexual pain), is associated with distress, and may interfere with other aspects of life. Among the different expressions of sexual difficulty, low desire—or loss of libido—is the most common, affecting up to half of women at some point in their lives.

The causes of sexual dysfunction in women are multifaceted and often unclear. In many women, the issues that contribute to ongoing sexual concerns may be quite different from the factors that originally provoked them. For example, the use of a medication that directly interferes with sexual response (such as an antidepressant) may have triggered the start of the difficulty, and then, over time, the woman's anxiety about whether or not she will respond sexually in the way she wants to may contribute to keeping the sexual dysfunction going. It is clear that sexual difficulties are associated with poor physical, emotional, and relationship well-being and are a major burden for many women.

My goal in writing this book is to bring the issue of low sexual desire in women into the open so that women feel less shame and are empowered to cultivate their feelings of sexual desire. In my own research to investigate effective treatments for women, I have focused on mindfulness meditation, an ancient Buddhist practice with a four-thousand-year history that involves paying attention compassionately and without judgment. I have been studying mindfulness as a potential treatment for sexual dysfunction in women since 2002, and over the years, many women, sex therapists, and physicians have asked me where they can learn more about this life-changing skill. This book is a response to those many requests, and I hope that the research findings you will learn about here inspire you to make mindfulness a part of your life. I have included many of the exercises that the women participating in our research* have taken part in, in the hope that you can make them a regular part of your daily life. The ideas and suggestions throughout this book are based not on any one individual's personal experience but rather on the feedback (formal and informal) from hundreds and perhaps thousands of women who found paying attention to be key for unlocking their sexual drive.

---

* Research is typically a team effort, and while this book is based on my direct experience of evaluating mindfulness as a therapeutic approach, you'll see that in places I refer to "we" or "our" when I'm talking about research, for example, that my team and I collaborated on.

1999—A LANDMARK YEAR

THE YEAR 1999 was one of notable events in the field of sexuality. That was the year Viagra was approved for the treatment of erectile dysfunction in Canada (it had already been approved in the United States in 1998), and the colossal ensuing media coverage led several experts to ask: "What about women?" Many speculated that it would be only a matter of time before Pfizer, the pharmaceutical company that owned Viagra, turned its attention to women. This seemed appropriate given that there were no approved medications for the treatment of sexual dysfunction in women, and Viagra was thought to be effective in women too.

That same year, I was searching for new research to embark upon as I began my doctorate degree in Clinical Psychology. After spending hundreds of hours over a half-dozen years in a small testing room injecting rats, operating on their organs (including their brains), exposing them to stress, watching their sexual behaviors, and ultimately euthanizing them, I was ready for a new population to study (and comfier testing quarters). Moreover, although the rat provided a useful model on which to test the effects of various experimental manipulations on sex, in the end, it provided only an incomplete picture of the higher-order cognitive processes, like emotion, thinking, and desire—all pivotal in the human experience of sex.

Also in 1999, a landmark study published in the *Journal of the American Medical Association* (JAMA) claimed that 43 percent of women and 31 percent of men experienced "sexual dysfunction." That nearly half of women could meet the criteria for a sexual dysfunction suggested that either there was a real problem inhibiting women's healthy sexual functioning or these rates of dysfunction were exaggerated. Nearly every major media outlet reiterated the JAMA paper's findings about women's sexual dysfunction, igniting anxiety among women that they might be suffering from "FSD"*—and inspiring sex scientists to probe deeper into just what was behind these high rates of sexual discontent in women.

Influenced by the 1999 publication and my feminist beliefs about the need for solid science aimed at understanding the sexual experiences of women, I launched a series of studies examining sexual arousal in women with and without sexual concerns. I invited women into a university laboratory and, using a tampon-shaped probe called a vaginal photoplethysmograph, which the women inserted into their vaginas, measured their physical sexual arousal responses to erotic films—totally in private.

The vaginal photoplethysmograph emits a beam of infrared light, and a sensor on the probe detects the amount of light scattered from the vaginal wall. The degree to which light is absorbed into the walls of the vagina reflects how much blood has congested in the area, which, in turn, provides an indirect measure of physical sexual arousal. (Of course, the amount of blood flow into the genital area may not relate to how aroused a woman says she is—a topic that will be explored more fully later.) Some of this research revealed differences between women with and without sexual difficulties when they were tested in this lab environment.

A notable influence on my research questions was the direct result of the hours I trained under Dr. Rosemary Basson,

---

* Although FSD, or female sexual dysfunction, is used regularly in the medical literature as referring to a particular condition, it is worth noting that FSD is an umbrella term that includes various sexual dysfunction diagnoses in women. As an imprecise diagnosis, it does not tell one whether the "dysfunction" pertains to motivation for sex, to the capacity for a physical sexual arousal response, or to pain with sex.

a physician and director at Vancouver's BC Centre for Sexual Medicine and a luminary in the study of women's sexuality. Basson listened intently to women's stories of their loss of sexual desire and how they mourned the spontaneous sexual desire of their youth. As her patients spoke, Basson started to draw a circle on her notepad using the following words: incentives for sex → sexual triggers → sexual arousal first → responsive sexual desire emerges → sexual satisfaction → greater incentive for sex (which closed the circle). She formulated a circular sexual response cycle (discussed in more detail in Chapter 4), which encouraged women to identify the factors that could elicit sexual arousal for them by inviting them to think about *why* they had sex, and also what types of triggers made them aroused. Basson helped women to appreciate that their sexual desire did not need to be present *before* a sexual encounter but could be cultivated *during* sexual activity. She helped thousands of women to feel normal* and empowered. Her innovative thinking about the responsive nature of sexual desire was key in my work exploring mindfulness as one way of eliciting women's sexual response and paying attention to it.

The years I spent with Basson, early in my career and in the decade since, convinced me that there was much variability in how women experienced and expressed their sexual desire and in the various triggers that could elicit a sexual response. Where women generally aligned was in their view that biomedical factors alone were rarely the underlying cause of their sexual complaints. Moreover, once they learned that sexual

---

* I am fully aware that the term "normal" can elicit negative reactions as it may imply that there are only two categories: normal and abnormal. However, the use of normal in this case (and throughout this book) is intended to mean common, expected, and entirely within the range of human experiences. Women themselves often use the word normal when they feel validated and understood in their sexuality.

desire could be ignited, and that it often emerged *after* they started a sexual encounter and experienced sexual arousal, they were keen to learn new skills to cultivate sexual desire naturally. They seemed to be asking us to teach them ways to tune in.

MY INTRODUCTION TO MINDFULNESS

"I FEEL ALIVE... fully connected... totally present. Nothing else in the world mattered." These were some of the phrases a sample of women from Seattle uttered when I interviewed them about their experiences of sexual desire. I was doing my postdoctoral fellowship with Dr. Julia Heiman at the University of Washington School of Medicine, and we wanted to know more about how women talked about sexual desire when they had it. The women told me stories about when, where, and how they felt sexual desire and opened a window onto their most private encounters. It is evident to me now—though it was not at the time—that these women were engaging mindfully during their pleasurable sexual encounters, and when they felt sexual desire, they were also fully in the moment—and certainly not thinking about to-do lists or whether they had run out of milk. Little did I realize that I was about to immerse myself in mindfulness training and that it would change everything I understood about sexual response in women.

I had begun an intensive therapy training program to learn dialectical behavior therapy (DBT), a skills-based treatment to address self-harm and suicidal behaviors. Patients in a DBT program receive a combination of individual weekly sessions with a therapist, in which they use problem solving to deal with the week's crises, and participate in a weekly skills group where they are taught specific problem-solving skills in interpersonal effectiveness, tolerance of distress, regulation of emotions, and mindfulness. The mindfulness practice involves remaining in the present moment, fully experiencing each negative sensation and emotion, and resisting the tendency to both think about the future or ruminate about the past and also fend off any negative feelings. Patients are taught that they can tolerate the distressing negative emotions of the present moment if they can learn to remain with them, riding each wave of seemingly intolerable feelings—even suicidal ones.

The mindfulness practice intrigued me—and puzzled me—the most, and I thought about Amanda*—a woman I was treating who went home each night after work, locked herself in her bathroom, and used her husband's razor blade to cut perfectly parallel lines in her wrist, an act that brought her relief as she watched the blood seep out. Cutting helped her deal with the intensely negative feelings she had toward her boss, her fear of losing her husband, and her belief that she had no close friends. Could teaching Amanda to pay attention to her negative thoughts, intense emotions, and impulse to cut her wrists actually reduce her nightly cutting ritual? I learned that teaching people like Amanda to pay attention to the present moment, to notice the details of the breath, and to "ride out" their in-the-moment urge to hurt themselves put them safely in the here-and-now. It was not the current moment that was unbearable to them; rather, it was future-oriented thoughts about having a life not worth living, a life of torment that would never come to an end, that made them feel hopeless and suicidal. There was safety and a sense of calm in the present moment, even if that included really intense negative feelings.

---

* All stories are based on actual patients, but names and details have been changed.

Observing suicidal clients "surf" their intense feelings with mindfulness and ground themselves in the present conveyed to me that mindfulness could be an effective way of putting people in touch with real sensations and shielding them from imagined or expected outcomes and scenarios. If all one had to do was pay attention, to tune in to the "truth" of present-moment bodily sensations and feelings, then it seemed to me that mindfulness was potentially a cure for the suffering experienced by so many people.

I had started reading about the emerging science of teaching meditation to patients with depression, anxiety, and chronic pain. New findings showed that mindfulness helped reduce stress and improve immune function in cancer survivors, and this translated into an improved quality of life. In my clinical practice, I was seeing gynecologic cancer survivors with sex-related problems. Many of these women had received surgical treatment to remove their infected organs (such as the cervix or uterus) or radiation therapy, which led to scar tissue and impairments in blood flow.

One day, a patient I will call Anya said to me, while fighting back tears, "I don't feel anything in my sexual parts. I want to have sex, but when we start, my body just doesn't cooperate. My genitals feel dead." Anya was one of many cancer survivors who said they did not notice any vaginal lubrication and felt no sexual arousal in their body. No pulsing. No tingling. No electricity. And yet, when they came into the sexual psycho-physiology laboratory at the University of Washington and we measured their vaginal blood flow response while they reclined and watched a series of short erotic films, the vaginal photo-plethysmograph recorded a strong genital blood flow response.

How could a robust genital response be happening without women noticing it? How could it be so different from men's experiences of having an erection, in which they invariably were aware of the erection and felt in the mood for sex? When men were tested in a similar lab setup (with a penile strain gauge—a rubber-band-like instrument placed over the flaccid penis that detects and measures an erection—instead of a vaginal probe), their erections tended to parallel how sexually aroused they reported feeling while watching porn. I wondered whether what we were observing in these women might be an example of the brain-body disconnect, where a physical response in the body is not registered in the person's mind, leaving her totally unaware that the physical response is happening. Could women be taught to pay attention to their bodies during sexual stimulation, and would this increase the brain-body communication in a way that might trigger sexual desire? Could mindfulness be a way of enhancing that connection?

I immersed myself in learning about mindfulness. First, to understand the origins of mindfulness meditation, I read *The Miracle of Mindfulness* by Thich Nhat Hanh, a Buddhist monk. Then I read the books of Jon Kabat-Zinn, an American molecular biologist who is credited with introducing mindfulness to the Western world through its applications to people living with chronic pain. In *Full Catastrophe Living: Using the Wisdom of Your Body and Mind to Face Stress, Pain, and Illness*, Kabat-Zinn describes the early formation of mindfulness-based stress reduction (MBSR), which he taught to patients with intractable pain at the University of Massachusetts Medical Center.

There was so much richness in how Kabat-Zinn wrote about mindfulness for chronic pain and so much relevance to the women with cancer and sexual dysfunction that I was treating. As I thought about the stories women shared with me when I asked them how they knew they felt sexual desire, it became evident to me that feeling sexual desire corresponded with being mindful. Maybe sexual desire was not even possible unless one was mindful. Perhaps some of the mindfulness exercises found to benefit patients with suicidal tendencies and chronic pain might also benefit women who had lost their sexual sensations. It seemed to be a perfect hypothesis that we could test.

THE BEGINNINGS OF
MINDFULNESS-BASED SEX THERAPY

GYNECOLOGIC ONCOLOGISTS AT the Seattle Cancer Care Alliance often saw women in their post-treatment follow-up appointments who had these problems, but they had very few treatment options to offer and were keen to collaborate with us. Dr. Heiman at the University of Washington, two of my clinical psychology supervisors, and I therefore cobbled together the skeleton of a three-session mindfulness-based program for gynecologic cancer survivors with sexual arousal problems.

Within a month, the cancer doctors had referred twenty-five women who had been treated with radical hysterectomy for early-stage cervical cancer to my study. During my telephone calls with the women before enrolling them in our study, I consistently heard comments such as, "My body has betrayed me—first by cancer, and now with a sexual dysfunction," accompanied by deep sadness and distress about the apparent loss. Most of the women I spoke with were young (under fifty) and not prepared to accept a sexless life. Although the prospect of losing their partners because of the sexual concerns brought on utter dread, many of them said they would "understand" if their partner left them for someone who still had the capacity to feel sexual. These women were motivated to take part in whatever treatment was available to them, even if it was something that had not yet been shown by science to work. Because what I had to offer them did not entail administering medications or hormones, they seemed open to participating in this experimental trial. Also, given the degree of their sex-related distress, many of them felt that they could not possibly be any worse off after this new experimental program.

The women came into my office, one by one, and we breathed together—slowly and with focus. I guided them to notice sensations in different parts of their body and to watch for the tendency for their minds to wander. The instructions were simple: pay attention, notice the dominant sensation and the smaller sensations that make up the dominant one, guide the mind back when it drifts, and so on. After completing this exercise with about two dozen women, we examined the women's responses and found that our brief mindfulness-based program helped this group of cervical cancer survivors to experience a significant increase in their levels of sexual desire and arousal. To our delight, they also reported a statistically significant reduction in sex-related distress and depressive symptoms, an increase in sexual satisfaction, and improvements in overall mental well-being.

After the pilot study, we repeated the study at the University of British Columbia with a larger sample of cancer survivors. Half the women waited a few months before beginning the mindfulness program so that we could measure what happens to their sexual response simply as a function of waiting to get into treatment. Whereas levels of sexual desire and arousal did not change during the months that the women waited to begin the program, participating in the mindfulness program led to the same significant improvements in sexual response and desire that women taking part in the pilot study had shown. It seemed to us that mindfulness was responsible for these improvements and that simply "waiting it out" did not lead to any improvements in their libidos.

Over the next several years, our team of collaborators expanded to include key experts in sexual medicine and mindfulness meditation in Vancouver, BC. My own personal practice in mindfulness continued as I became part of a group of therapists who met monthly to deepen our own experience with meditation under the careful guidance of teachers. Our research team received funding from the Canadian Institutes of Health Research to examine mindfulness in a variety of different populations of women with sexual concerns as well as women with genital pain (discussed later in this book). The women participating in our program provided rich feedback, which strengthened our program, and their feedback shaped the treatment manuals that guided our exercises. Now, a dozen years later, mindfulness has been accepted as an important treatment option for women with sexual dysfunction, and experts around the world are seeking their own formal training in mindfulness in hopes of sharing these skills with their patients.

This book is intended for women of all ethnic backgrounds, cultures, ages, sociocultural positions, genders, bodies, orientations, and relationship statuses. Whether you are struggling with a sexual difficulty such as low libido or lack of orgasm or you simply want to enhance your sex life, I hope that the simple practice of paying attention, nonjudgmentally, moment by moment, will cultivate sexual desire and a new awareness of sexual arousal for you.

CHAPTER 1

SEX IN A
MULTITASKING WORLD

Ultimately, I see mindfulness as a love affair—with life,
with reality and imagination, with the beauty of your own being, with
your heart and body and mind, and with the world.

JON KABAT-ZINN, *Mindfulness for Beginners: Reclaiming*
the Present Moment—and Your Life

I N MOST RESPECTS, Shelina was a typical forty-eight-year-old married woman and mother of two. She had a thriving career as the lead realtor at her firm, her teenage children were well adjusted and confident, and she and her husband, Akmal, had a rich circle of friends and social activities. However, Shelina had a secret she could not share. Inside, she felt broken. The fire that she once felt when gazing at her partner was now a dull flicker. She longed for the physical cravings she used to experience for sex that had been replaced by an orchestrated plan and predictable outcome.

During her weekly sexual encounters, which were planned for Friday nights between 11:00 and 11:15 pm, she deliberately avoided the foreplay she used to enjoy. No more kissing, touching, or caressing. She would zone out while Akmal touched her—thinking about plans for the next day and engaging very little with her body—prompting him to move directly to sexual intercourse, which she found unrewarding. And the less gratifying that sex had become, the more her sexual motivation had diminished to the point where she debated about whether she should concede to her partner's requests. All other facets of Shelina's relationship were "perfect" by her estimation, so her lack of desire for Akmal mystified her. She was convinced that she had a deep-seated psychological obstruction that was preventing her from feeling desire. And despite her seeing a few well-qualified sex therapists over the years, Shelina's sexual desire would not revive.

So many women can relate to Shelina's dilemma. She adores her partner, but the unrewarding nature of sex has extinguished her sexual desire. And the more she avoids physical contact, the less likely her body will remember what arousal cues are, making it even more difficult for her to become sexually excited. She is stuck in a vicious cycle and does not know how to break it. For some women, this picture of sexual dissatisfaction persists throughout their lives.

Despite the societal obsession with sexuality and the prevailing belief that sex is a universally powerful and energizing force, sexual difficulties are immensely prevalent. Many women around the world and across ages have difficulty reaching orgasm. Insufficient lubrication affects not just postmenopausal or breastfeeding women but women of all ages, regardless of their hormonal status. Like Shelina, many women find that sex is often unrewarding. "This doesn't feel pleasurable...it feels as though my partner is touching my elbow" is a common complaint uttered by many women, as erotic feelings become replaced with neutral or even negative feelings. Penetration is uncomfortable or even painful for some. And the motivation for sex is drastically reduced, or simply not there for countless women.

THE SCIENTIFIC EVIDENCE

TO SEX THERAPISTS or sexual medicine clinicians who devote their time to helping women with these complaints, it is no surprise that such concerns are very common—in fact, they are much more common than most people might think. In 1999, soon after Viagra's approval in 1998, the *Journal of the American Medical Association* (JAMA) published a study titled "Sexual Dysfunction in the United States: Prevalence and Predictors," which was based on the large National Health and Social Life Survey. In this study, three thousand American women and men between the ages of eighteen and fifty-nine took part in a face-to-face interview with a trained researcher. They were asked in detail about their sexual functioning, and they had to indicate whether any of the following had been a problem in the past twelve months: lack of desire for sex, arousal difficulties (defined as erection problems in men and lubrication difficulties in women), difficulty achieving orgasm, anxiety about sexual performance, climaxing or ejaculating too quickly, physical pain during intercourse, or not finding sex pleasurable. The researchers limited their analyses to respondents who reported having been sexually active with at least one partner in the previous year.

Among women, the most common sexual complaint was a lack of sexual interest, which was endorsed by 32 percent of the youngest age group (eighteen to twenty-nine years old) and 27 percent of the oldest age group (fifty to fifty-nine years old). An inability to reach orgasm was also very common, and more so among younger women than older women. Not finding sex pleasurable was nearly twice as common in the youngest age group as in the oldest age group—challenging societal beliefs that youthful sex is always pleasurable and rewarding. Experiencing pain during sex affected one in every five women and has been the focus of much scientific research over the past decade. (This topic is covered in detail in Chapter 9.) Anxiety about performance during sex was also very common among younger women.

The only sexual concern found to increase in prevalence with age was trouble lubricating, which affected one in five young women and one in four older women. When the researchers examined the prevalence of any type of sexual concern, a total of 43 percent of the women participants were found to have a sexual dysfunction, compared with 31 percent of the men. In other words, nearly half of American women were labeled as having a sexual dysfunction of some type.

A few years later, Pfizer, the drug-giant makers of Viagra, sponsored an international study that compared the rates of sexual difficulties in men and women across different regions of the world. The Global Study of Sexual Attitudes and Behaviors analyzed the data from nearly twenty thousand women and men aged forty to eighty, living in twenty-nine countries, who had been sexually active at least once over the previous year. Using a more stringent definition of sexual difficulty, the study team analyzed the frequency of sexual difficulties that were at least sometimes occurring over a two-month period in the past year. Lack of sexual interest was still the most frequent sexual complaint in women, affecting one out of every two to four women, depending on the region of the world they lived in. Lack of interest was less common in men, affecting 12 to 28 percent of men globally. Rates of sexual problems related to orgasm, arousal, and pleasure were similar to those in the JAMA study, and concerns were consistently higher in East Asian and Middle Eastern countries than in other countries. In fact, the study found quite marked cross-cultural differences in the prevalence of sexual concerns by world region. Across the twenty-nine countries in the study, women living in North Africa and the Middle East (Algeria, Egypt, Morocco, and Turkey), East Asia (China, Hong Kong, Japan, Korea, and Taiwan), and Southeast Asia (Indonesia, Malaysia, Philippines, Singapore, and Thailand) were significantly more likely to experience problems with sexual interest, inability to reach orgasm, painful sex, not finding sex pleasurable, and difficulties with lubrication.

Although the reasons behind the higher rates in these regions of the world were not a topic of the study, the researchers speculated that cultural attitudes about sexuality, particularly among women, could be at least partially responsible.

One of the largest sex surveys is the National Survey of Sexual Attitudes and Lifestyles (NATSAL), which has been carried out three times between 1990 and 2012 in Britain. The NATSAL used a probability sampling method, which means that it aimed to obtain a representative sample of British residents between the ages of sixteen and seventy-four. A total of 15,162 men and women were interviewed in depth about many aspects of their sexual health, behaviors, and beliefs. A subset of participants also provided hormone samples via saliva, urine samples, or vaginal smears. Because the NATSAL was carried out three times over twenty-two years, it allowed the research team to examine trends in sexual practices over time. Moreover, the scope of the sample and the rigorous approach the research team used to obtain a representative sample mean that the NATSAL data are considered to be quite a valid reflection of current sex practices, beliefs, and behaviors (in Western societies).

The NATSAL asked about a broad array of different sexual problems and, in addition, aspects of participants' relationships such as whether the couple communicated about sex, and whether respondents felt that they and their partner had differing levels of sexual desire. Mirroring the findings from the earlier large-scale studies, lack of interest in sex was the most common sexual difficulty—it affected one-third of the women, and was twice as common in women as it was in men.

Across the different sexual complaints, 51 percent of the women reported at least one sexual concern lasting three months or longer over the previous year. Wow—half of women reporting a sexual concern? These figures appear to be higher than in earlier large studies and introduce the question of whether the rates of sexual dysfunction in women are rising, even just over the past decade.

Do these extremely high rates of sexual difficulties mean that sex therapists are being inundated with clients? Not exactly. This is because not all women who report a sexual difficulty are bothered by it. In fact, the NATSAL found that 10 percent of the women were distressed because of sex, but that less than 20 percent of them sought help or advice about sex and that they were much more likely to consult the Internet for sexual advice than to seek guidance from a qualified professional. In other words, only a subset of women with sexual difficulties and low sexual desire are distressed about those sexual problems, and only a fraction of women with low desire and distress are likely to seek help. Of course, it may also be that embarrassment contributes to the low rates of seeking help given that large studies find that individuals are very reluctant to talk about sexual problems with even their close friends.

As a sex therapist and researcher, I am fascinated by this statistic. Is it because addressing sexual problems with a health-care provider can be embarrassing and awkward, so women adapt by "learning to live with it"? Is it that the sexual difficulties are problems only for a woman's partner but not for her? A more recent North American study, led out of the University of Massachusetts and published in 2008, of thirty thousand women found similar rates of overall sexual difficulty and identified low libido as the most common complaint. This study also looked more deeply at the issue of distress about sex and speculated that other significant medical issues among the older women may have mitigated some of the distress associated with their sexual problems—in other words, it allowed for the possibility that some of the women had bigger health issues on their mind than their sexual problems.

So, sexual difficulties are common. Very common. And low sexual desire, in particular, is consistently the most common sex-related concern that women report, whether they are from North or South America, Europe, Australia, or Asia. Are sexual problems becoming more prevalent? Why do they appear to affect women more than men? Are there causes of sexual difficulty in women that are a by-product of our current culture and the messages that women are bombarded with to be, look, act, and think a certain way? And to what extent can such sexual difficulties be reversed or even stopped? Research has only begun to address these questions in a systematic way, and answers to most of them are still elusive.

Since the British NATSAL study was carried out three times between 1990 and 2012, we can at least answer the question of whether sexual difficulties have become more or less prevalent with time. Low desire in men was more common in the 2010–2012 wave than in the first wave, twenty years earlier. Also interesting was the change in sexual frequency and practices across the three waves of NATSAL. How often people were having sex decreased from 6.3 episodes per month in 2001 to 4.8 episodes per month in 2012. International headlines such as "Not tonight, darling: Why is Britain having less sex?" and "It's not just you. Americans are having less sex" garnered a lot of attention and caused members of the public to reflect on their own sex lives. What is happening in contemporary society that is causing people to not only have less sex but also be less interested in sex? Is this a passing fad or a trend that is expected to increase in the future?

POSSIBLE CAUSES OF LOW SEXUAL DESIRE

IN A 2008 North American study, depression was found to double the odds of a person having distressing low sexual desire. In other words, women experiencing depression were twice as likely as women with normal mood to have low sexual desire and to be distressed by it. Every survey assessing the prevalence of low desire, regardless of where that survey was carried out, identifies depression as a major risk factor for low desire. Because of this, and because of how often I see low desire along with low mood among my clients, I will revisit the role of depression in more depth later.

Since not every woman who participated in these large-scale national studies experiences a sexual problem, or loses her sexual desire, you might be wondering: Why are some people more vulnerable to developing a sexual dysfunction than others? Or: Will I be one of those who is in danger of losing my libido? Or maybe even: Why am I one of those women struggling with absent libido?

Let's look at Susan and Juanita. Both are forty-five-year-old heterosexual women who work full-time and have two children. Both women are in relatively good health, drink alcohol only socially, and do not use medications. Susan and Juanita both had limited sex education at school and have never suffered any form of sexual abuse or coercion. Susan has had low sexual desire for most of her adult life, has never had a sexual fantasy, and has never initiated sex in any of her past relationships. Juanita, on the other hand, looks forward to sex, initiates sex regularly with her husband, and even plans sexual encounters (e.g., she will leave a note in her husband's bag inviting him to a "date night" that night). How could two women who superficially have so much in common have such disparate experiences of sexual desire?

Scientists have been intrigued by this question for a long time and have used the existing large population-based surveys to try to identify characteristics of people that might make them more vulnerable to developing a sexual dysfunction. For instance, unmarried American women in the National Health and Social Life Survey were more likely to have problems with orgasm and sexual anxiety than were married women. Women who had not graduated from high school were twice as likely to have low desire, problems with orgasm, sexual pain, and sex-related anxiety as women with a college-level education. Health-related factors found to increase the odds of experiencing a sexual problem for women included low mood and anxiety, as well as experiencing daily stress (much more will be said about this later); on a physical level, urinary tract symptoms caused pain and affected arousal in women. Nearly half of those with poor sexual function had symptoms of depression, and 70 percent had fair to very bad health. Being unemployed also increased the odds of having a sexual problem.

Susan and Juanita share many characteristics, but they also differ in one particular characteristic that turns out to be very important for whether one develops a sexual problem or not: beliefs about sex. Susan believes that sex has a role in reproduction but is a frivolous and self-indulgent activity when pursued for pleasure. She resists the thought that sex can be fun, and she shuns her partner for suggesting that it could be a shared leisure activity. After her own mother transitioned through menopause and struggled with debilitating hot flashes, night sweats, difficulty concentrating, and depression, Susan sees aging as the end of any remaining interest in sexual activity.

In contrast, Juanita believes that sex is a form of communication between her and her partner and a unique form of expression that she does not share with anyone else. She has a broad list of reasons for why she engages in sex, including that it is fun, she delights in orgasms, sex can help her relax and get to sleep, and it fortifies intimacy in her relationship. Juanita believes that she can have different incentives for sex at different times, and she sees sex as playing an important role in her life as she ages, particularly when she and her husband retire and have more free time.

It turns out that whether you believe sex is important or not, and how strongly you hold on to some of the prevailing myths about age and sex, can predict whether you will develop a sexual concern or not. Research shows that women who believe that age diminishes sexual desire and sexual activity are twice as likely to experience low sexual desire as women who do not hold this belief. What's more, women who had lost hope about the future of their relationship were two to three times as likely to experience sexual pain and low sexual desire as women who still felt hopeful about their relationships.

Our beliefs about sex are greatly influenced by where we receive our sex education and how much of it we receive. It will probably come as no surprise that our sexual health behaviors and concerns as adults are influenced in part by how our sex education was delivered and by whom. Ideally, sex education would be delivered by trained professionals in schools as part of the standard curriculum. In the third wave of the British NATSAL study, people who reported that they received sex education primarily from school tended to be older when they started having sex and were subsequently less likely to engage in unsafe sex and less likely to have a range of other negative sexual health outcomes, including less likelihood of becoming the victim of sexual assault, fewer occurrences of a sexually transmitted infection, and less distress about sex. In other words, school-integrated sex education programs that are not based on an "abstinence-only" model contribute to healthier sexuality later on. Although the findings strongly support the benefits of providing sex education (ideally through a combination of parents and school), sex education programs vary widely in quality across cities, regions, and countries. Most programs lack evidence-based information, and many focus on scare tactics ("If you have sex, you will certainly get pregnant") and gross generalizations that do not consider the wide variability of people, preferences, and experiences. Almost no school-based sex education programs address sexual pleasure.

Most young people do not have enough information about sex (such as how to protect against sexually transmitted infections and how to prevent pregnancy) when they become sexually active, and surveys show that they want more information. It is well known that many of the sex-related beliefs people hold as adults stem from our early experiences in life, including early formal sex education, sexual experiences we had, and sexual attitudes and behavior we observed in those around us. Did you grow up in a home where you could ask questions about sexuality? Did your parents and other adults close to you express love and affection? Did you have someone to turn to when you were confused about your feelings for a classmate and about what those feelings meant?

I am always struck by the number of women I speak with who report feeling embarrassed and anxious about masturbation. It saddens me. When I ask them why they are embarrassed about an activity that typically occurs alone and in total privacy, they usually tell a story about an earlier time in their life when they had a negative experience related to it. Perhaps they were made to believe that it would make hair grow on their hands. Maybe they were told that they would no longer be a virgin if they masturbated. Or maybe, as is the case for so many women, someone walked in on them while they were masturbating and they were humiliated and horrified. "This makes no sense to me as a mature, adult woman," I have heard women say countless times. "But, emotionally, I feel the same embarrassment, anxiety, and awkwardness about masturbation as I did when I was young." Again, we are reminded that who we are sexually as adults is, in part, directly affected by our early life experiences.

Low sexual desire is very common in all women, not only in older women. The high rates of low desire in young women are surprising to many and directly challenge the prevailing belief that low desire is associated with old age. In fact, younger women are found to have more distress than older women about their lack of libido. Adolescent women, too, can experience low sexual desire, and a large body of research by Canadian researchers led by Dr. Lucia O'Sullivan shows that low sexual desire affects one-quarter of women in the sixteen-to-twenty-one age range. Why are rates of sexual problems so high among adolescents? The researchers speculated that the "sexual double standard" may have been at play—teaching women to be sexually passive and acquiesce to a man's sexual solicitations and thereby not cultivating her sense of sexual autonomy and agency. Of course, lack of sexual experience and anxiety leading to unfulfilling encounters may also explain the high prevalence of low desire among adolescent women.

If heart disease, asthma, or diabetes affected so many people, including young people, there would be an immediate surge in resources made available to assess, diagnose, treat, and research these conditions to find out why they are so common in our youth. But problems related to sexual health or sexual response do not elicit the same sense of urgency or mobilization of resources. Women experience a great degree of shame about their sexual concerns, believing that they "should" want sex more, they "should" enjoy sex like everyone else they know does, and they "should" know what they want sexually and how to ask for it. Unfortunately, women are often oblivious to the fact that some of the women they believe are enjoying frequent and passionate sex are actually secretly experiencing a similar set of sexual problems. Too often, women "should" themselves ruthlessly, compounding their struggles and making themselves feel unwhole.

Not all health-care providers, including primary care physicians, receive training in how to thoroughly assess sexual response and in the treatment of sexual concerns. As a result, even when a woman reaches out to her family doctor for help, she may be met with embarrassment, more questions than answers, or a simple "I don't know." Women are thus often left to deal with their concerns on their own. Many seek advice through Internet discussion groups, which can help women feel they are not alone, but the information shared is not regulated and may not meet the test of scientific rigor and therefore may not lead to any meaningful improvements.

THE ROLE OF DEPRESSION AND STRESS

WE HAVE LEARNED much about the role of depression in sexual dysfunction, and we are learning more about the effects of stress and daily challenges. It has long been known that the loss of a loved one, a traumatic accident, or a major life change such as a divorce or a move to a new city can make people vulnerable to depression. We now know that daily life events can also add up to create extreme levels of stress for many people. The hamster wheel of work, domestic life, parenting, financial struggles, health issues, relationship conflict, and feeling like we are being pulled in a multitude of directions throughout the day can cause many of us to feel chronically stressed as well as detached from partners, friends, and our larger social network. Consider Cynthia's situation.

Cynthia—a fifty-six-year-old woman in a bright, multi-colored blouse, pleated gray trousers, and trendy wedged sandals—sat across from me on the blue suede sofa of my office. Within the first five minutes of our meeting, after I had asked what brought her to see me today, she began to sob, followed by repeated apologies for sobbing, which led, predictably, to more tears. "My desire has completely vanished," she said through tears.

As she shared her story, it became evident that Cynthia's work stress contributed a lot to her loss of sexual desire. She had been a psychiatric nurse for twenty-five years, working in a very emotionally demanding but rewarding job in an inpatient unit at a major hospital. She also led the adolescent psychiatric program that designed and delivered coping strategies to suicidal teens who were hospitalized on a short-term basis until their suicidal thoughts became less intense. She was very good at her job and derived much personal satisfaction from improving the lives of the hundreds of young people she had worked with over the years. But when one of the medical directors told her that as a nonphysician she could not make decisions about whether or not a patient should be discharged from the hospital, Cynthia abruptly quit her job. She felt that the director's statement undermined all her years of experience of working with troubled teens, and, in fact, she had been part of the team that made decisions about patients' discharge for two decades, since she had both the experience and the insight to be trusted to make such decisions.

That evening Cynthia started looking for another job. Within a week she had secured a job at a school, where her role was to provide counseling to students. She found the students seeking her guidance to be resistant to her suggestions and even rude to her. Because the parents believed that technology upgrades were a more pressing need than a school counselor, they were aloof toward her, and she felt that she did not fit in with the tight-knit staff.

She began to regret her impulsive decision to quit her former job. She knew that she could not go back to the inpatient unit, and she believed she now had a "bad reputation" as a loose cannon. She also felt guilty for leaving those teens on the inpatient unit. She worried about whether they would receive the kind, compassionate, and validating support from the new staff member who had replaced her—someone who was three decades her junior. She was faced with the perceived realization that she had abandoned those teens, and she felt responsible for their well-being in the face of their acute suicidal tendencies. As her regret, guilt, and anxiety intensified, so did her unhappiness in her new job. She could not find any joy in school counseling, and she doubted whether any of the students found her advice useful.

After eight months, Cynthia found herself in a full-blown depression. She had stopped socializing with her friends and attending her ballroom dancing group, which she had previously loved. Her energy level was low, and despite sleeping ten hours a night, she woke up exhausted. Cynthia's marriage started to suffer as well. Although she and her husband had had ups and downs throughout their thirty-year relationship, they had always been able to overcome conflict through excellent communication. Now Cynthia began to shut out her husband, saying to him, "What is the point in talking about this? It's not going to resolve the situation." Such catastrophic thinking was not like Cynthia, who, as a professional counselor, would encourage her clients to challenge such ways of thinking. She simply could not do so herself in the face of her active depression.

Cynthia had always enjoyed sex. She was easily aroused and regularly reached orgasm during sex, and she loved the feelings of pleasure that surged through her body. Since the onset of her depression, however, sex had become infrequent. In the span of a year, Cynthia went from having sex once or twice a week to only once in the past three months. Furthermore, she did not miss it. Cynthia interpreted her loss of desire as yet another failure on her part and suggested to her husband that he might consider seeing a sex worker, given that she could not imagine ever wanting to have sex again.

Cynthia's experience is one that I regularly encounter in my clinical practice and one that is well known to all sex therapists. Mental health, anxiety, and stress are major exterminators of sexual desire and arousal in women. Women with low desire are far more likely to experience symptoms of depression or a full-blown depressive disorder like Cynthia's than women who do not have concerns about their sexual desire. In a 2003 study of one thousand American women aged twenty to sixty-five, the strongest predictor of sex-related distress was mood and emotional well-being (as well as the quality of the relationship). And although an unsatisfying sex life undoubtedly contributes to unhappiness, it is likely that low mood directly disrupts sexuality. Science reveals that a negative mood has a much greater effect on sex than physiological factors, such as vaginal lubrication. A hallmark feature of depression is apathy—or a generalized lack of interest in activities that one formerly found enjoyable. Cynthia experienced this as a loss of interest in ballroom dancing, an activity that she previously relished. Sex is one of the previously enjoyable activities that people who are depressed typically lose motivation for. The combination of apathy, daily stress, and social withdrawal can be difficult to penetrate, and loss of sexual desire may become chronic, as it had for Cynthia and other women like her.

OUR STRESSED-OUT SOCIETY

ACCORDING TO THE Stress in America Survey, which has been carried out by the American Psychological Association annually since 2007, up to one-third of Americans have reported extreme stress in their daily lives since 2013. The main sources of stress are money, work, and the economy, and when asked about what types of stress they anticipate in the years to come, personal health and the health of loved ones rose to the top. Over half of those surveyed stated that they would like more emotional support to deal with daily stress. Increasingly, we rely on technological advances to accomplish the never-ending list of tasks on our to-do list and "multitask." Being "able" to eat, respond to emails, surf the Internet, check Facebook, and help a child with homework all at the same time makes many of us feel proficient, and we take pride in balancing all these different activities at the same time. How many times have you responded to the question "How are you?" with "I'm so busy!" Being busy is the norm, and if you are not busy, what are you?

But research suggests that the daily grind can be extremely stressful for many of us, and multitasking may contribute to our feeling that we cannot get our head above water. If we are doing more and juggling multiple tasks on our to-do list at the same time, why do we perpetually feel like we are falling behind? Neuroscientists have shown that multitasking may not be as productive as we think it is, and the term itself is a misnomer, because we don't actually multitask, or complete multiple tasks at the same time. We shift between tasks in rapid serial progression. This rapid shifting carries a "cognitive load," or certain amount of mental effort, and each "switch" is associated with a cost in our brain's processing ability and speed. Research sponsored by Hewlett-Packard assigned workers to carry out mentally demanding tests in two environments—one in which all distracting devices were removed, and one in which phones were left on and email alerts were audible. The findings indicate that the presence of phones and other electronic devices that issued, for example, email alerts, caused significant distraction, which amounted to about the same as a 10-point drop in IQ. The author referred to this phenomenon as "infomania." Along with the drop in IQ, women self-reported a striking increase in how much stress they felt during this task.

Understanding the role and function of the hormone cortisol is key to understanding why stress is so destructive. When you are feeling stressed, the hypothalamus releases a hormone called corticotropin-releasing hormone (CRH). (Exercise and sleep-wake cycles can also trigger the release of CRH.) CRH then acts on the anterior pituitary, in another part of the brain, to release adrenocorticotropic hormone (ACTH), which signals the adrenal glands to release cortisol. Cortisol's main function is to regulate a range of functions in the body, including immune responses and reactions to stress. In healthy people, cortisol rises rapidly when you wake up and then gradually falls over the course of the day, with a very distinct and sharp rise within 30 minutes of waking followed by a decrease, known as the cortisol awakening response. Separate from the decline in cortisol levels from morning to night, this cortisol awakening response is controlled by different brain regions involved in awakening. Stress can impair both the morning to night drop in cortisol, and also the cortisol awakening response. The blunting of this high-to-low slope in cortisol—most commonly, when cortisol remains high throughout the day—has been associated with several negative health conditions, including obesity, cardiovascular problems, smoking relapse, and inability to respond effectively to stressors. Thus, in humans, it is desirable to have a decline in cortisol from high in the morning to low at night.

In small doses (or in response to single-event stressors such as witnessing a car accident or a daring ski down a black diamond run), cortisol helps regulate many of the systems of the body to maintain homeostasis, or balance. In this situation, cortisol mobilizes a person (or an animal) to adapt or react to a stressful situation. However, in high doses, which occur with chronic, daily stress, the high-to-low cortisol slope becomes blunted. The stress response system becomes maladaptive and does not allow the organism to adapt to its environment, which means that the body is unable to return to a state of balance and instead remains in a state of "fight or flight." In animal studies, a prolonged stress response has been found to impair parts of the brain involved in learning and memory, such as the hippocampus. The same damage is thought to occur in humans.

In addition to our tendency to multitask, which may fuel our feelings of stress, it seems that we are not very good at either managing stress or preventing it. According to the Stress in America Survey, Americans tend to choose sedentary activities as a means of stress management, with listening to music, reading, and napping being cited as some of the most common ways people relieve stress. The symptoms of stress most often described include irritability or anger, feeling nervous or anxious, feeling tired, feeling sad, and lacking energy. Lack of time was cited as both a major contributor to stress and a major barrier to stress-reduction. Paradoxically, our multitasking tendencies and increased capacity to be in multiple places at the same time (albeit virtually) have not saved us time. And this may contribute to our feeling more stressed than ever before.

So, how are dealing with never-ending to-do lists, floundering in a sea of tasks, and feeling the burden of daily challenges relevant to sexuality? It turns out that they are implicated in the loss of desire for sex in particular. If our brains are perpetually engaged in multitasking, as we continually attend to numerous competing demands on our attention, we actually spend very little time living in the present moment. We vacillate between thinking about the future (planning, worrying, strategizing) and living in the past (replaying scenes, ruminating over conversations, mourning missed opportunities). We spend far more time living outside of the present moment than in the present moment.

Brain-imaging studies show that distraction and inattention impair our ability to attend to and process sexual cues. Even in a highly sexually arousing situation, our brains may not be paying attention to sexual triggers that are necessary to elicit a sexual response, such as viewing an erotic scene in a movie or detecting the flirtatious gaze of a potential partner. It is as if the body is present but the mind is elsewhere—lost in thoughts, memories, or plans.

My bet is that most, or perhaps all, of the readers of this book have experienced at least one situation in which stress suppressed their sexual desire. In fact, it is likely that we are hardwired to respond this way as a result of our evolutionary history. The fight or flight response, which is triggered when we are faced with a stressor, activates our sympathetic nervous system—the branch of our brain that has evolved over time to help us cope in an adaptive way to serious life stressors. Blood gets shunted to our major muscles to mobilize us to fight or flee. However, the physiological changes that take place when we are under stress backfire when stress is chronic. Remember Cynthia and her situation in which she felt stressed day after day, with no letting up? It is likely that her muscles were constantly tense, that she experienced changes in blood flow— such as the routing of blood flow to the major muscles and away from her periphery to allow for her to take flight—and that cortisol was being secreted at high levels all day long without the normal return to a baseline state in the first half of the night. Cynthia's body was reacting to her stressful work situation and preparing to engage in physical combat or sprint away from the scene. Over the many months that Cynthia's mood dipped and her feelings of stress intensified, all of these physiological changes coalesced to interfere with her body's ability to become sexually aroused. As a result, her motivation for sex and her feelings of pleasure during sex were dampened.

If you can relate somewhat to Cynthia's situation, or perhaps find yourself challenged by a never-ending to-do list and its devastating dampening effects on desire, then join me as we explore what you can do to make sex fabulous and fulfilling again.

CHAPTER 2

SEEKING SEXUAL ECSTASY–FROM THE COUCH TO THE BRAIN DRUG

*Defining the essence of sexuality as a specific sequence
of psychophysiological changes promotes biological reductionism.
Biological reductionism not only separates genital sexual
performance from personalities, relationships, conduct, context, and
values, it overvalues the former at the expense of the latter.*

LEONORE TIEFER, "Historic, Scientific, Clinical and
Feminist Criticisms of 'The Human Sexual Response Cycle' Model,"
Annual Review of Sex Research

A T FIFTY-SEVEN YEARS of age, Joanna felt that the time had come for her to prioritize her own health. As the only child of two elderly parents with multiple health conditions, Joanna had never experienced the carefree youth that her friends had. After school she would have to rush home to care for her father, who had multiple sclerosis, while her mother, who herself experienced chronic daily pains in her wrist and knee joints, worked two jobs to pay his medical bills.

While Joanna's friends were at the park playing hopscotch or hide-and-seek, she would be tending to her father's physical needs, measuring out his medications, and doing all of the household chores. She was not like other ten-year-olds: she would take a bus across town once a week to grocery shop, and she would deposit her mother's paycheck at the bank on her own. Joanna never resented her parents for the amount of responsibility she had because this was "normal" for her. Joanna became known as "Mini-mommy" among her peers, who knew her as the reliable person who could always be counted on.

Joanna was popular among the boys in high school because of her kindness and her reputation for always wanting to help people. She had her first boyfriend in college, and they married when Joanna was twenty-two years old. Her giving nature made her a natural for a career in nursing, which she pursued even as she raised her four children.

Although Joanna was devoted to her husband, her sex life was never very rewarding. She was unaware of how other women experienced sex, however, because the topic was quite private for her. It was not until she was fifty years old and her children began to reveal aspects of their own sexuality and sexual experiences that Joanna realized sex had never been satisfying. Her main motivation for sex with her husband was the same as it had always been: "because he needs sex." Her own pleasure and emotional needs had never been a motivation for her. She had not experienced orgasm, and in fact, even though she was a nurse and was familiar with the human body, she was not quite sure about her own sexual anatomy and did not know where to stimulate herself to elicit orgasm.

When she opened up to her two daughters about this, she realized that by wanting to please others and prioritizing her husband's needs, she had never taken pleasure in the recreational aspects of sex. Her sexual self-esteem—that is, her confidence in knowing who she was as a sexual woman—was very low, if not completely absent. The notion of initiating sex for her own pursuit of pleasure was foreign to her. As she reflected on her lifelong tendency to put other people's needs before her own, she gained insight into her current situation. But she also became increasingly distressed about her sexuality and her lack of agency, and she started to resent her husband.

At the suggestion of one of her daughters, Joanna enlisted the help of a skilled sex therapist, who provided her with the educational information she had never received earlier in life on women's sexual desire and talked about the multiple different motivations women have for engaging in sex. In addition to wanting to please a partner, women offer dozens (in fact, hundreds) of unique reasons why they initiate sex or are receptive to sex that is initiated by a partner. Their reasons run the gamut: to express love, celebrate a special holiday, share an emotional closeness, manage a relationship, or experience sexual gratification. Together with her sex therapist, Joanna also considered her selfless nature and the fact that she had never asked for what she wanted or needed—both nonsexually and, especially, sexually. Although she was well loved because of this trait, it was an obstacle to her pursuit of sexual pleasure.

Eventually, she started to become more sexually assertive and to pay attention to her own sensations during sex instead of focusing on her husband's satisfaction and happiness. For the first time in her life, and after almost four decades of formulaic sexual behavior with the same partner, Joanna began to feel sexual desire. And it felt good.

FREUD AND THE FIVE STAGES
OF PSYCHOSEXUAL DEVELOPMENT

IF JOANNA HAD been seeking treatment in the late nineteenth century, it is likely that her therapy would have lasted for years and focused on her stalled psychosexual development. In the early history of sex therapy, psychoanalysis was targeted at the unconscious mind and women's libido. Freud, known by many as the father of psychoanalysis, had a theory of psychosexual development based on the idea that each of us is born with an instinctual libido which, as we mature, undergoes five stages of development, each corresponding to a different type of behavior. He identified the stages of psychosexual development as oral, anal, phallic, latent, and genital. Each of the body locations (except at the latent stage) was thought to be the focus of one's libidinous drive. If one became fixated at any stage without maturing to the next one, certain negative psychological and sexual outcomes were inevitable. For example, fixation at the oral stage meant that an individual would become obsessed with oral stimulation, such as nail biting or oral sex. Fixation at the second, anal, stage could lead one to be "anally retentive" and have an obsessive need for tidiness and order or to be "anally expulsive" and behave recklessly and carelessly.

Freud believed that a woman's inability to have vaginal orgasms during sexual intercourse and her reliance on clitoral stimulation to experience orgasm was a sign of psychosexual immaturity and failure to develop past the third stage, the phallic stage—the stage at which one's libido is focused on one's own genitals. Freud believed that immature women could only experience orgasms through clitoral stimulation and that true sexual maturity was reached only when women "transferred" the locus of orgasmic release from the clitoris to the vagina.

During the fourth stage, the latency stage, not much sexual development occurs, but rather, the child's supposed sex drive toward their parents is transferred to same-sex friends. It is also a stage of developing the sense of self. In the fifth, or genital, stage, the individual develops sexual feelings for individuals outside of the family and shifts from solitary gratification-driven sexual activity to dyadic and emotional sex. Fixation at the genital stage of psychosexual development can give rise to extreme self-love, otherwise known as narcissism. Psychoanalytic treatment was focused on resolving stunted areas of psychosexual development by identifying conflicts between conscious and unconscious forces, and by using catharsis, which involved bringing deeply buried emotions to the surface, often by asking patients to recollect a traumatic event. Although psychoanalysis has been heavily criticized over the decades for lacking scientific rigor, some sex therapists continue to rely on it to address sexual concerns—New York City is home to many modern-day psychoanalysts who focus on addressing sexual problems.

The neo-Freudians who succeeded Freud categorized all sexual dysfunctions in women under the umbrella term "frigidity," which included an inability to have a vaginal orgasm. The desire for clitoral stimulation was deemed pathological and was associated with neurosis and social isolation. During the first half of the twentieth century, feminists and women who were attracted to women were also deemed pathological. Sexual problems were brought into the limelight because of their interference with women's "marital obligations." Problems in women's sexual desire—either too much or too little of it—were viewed through the lens of pathology, with women assumed to be not adhering to the norms of femininity.

Much of the focus of the sex therapists in the neo-Freudian

era was on helping women deal with the "trauma of the wedding night," when women would experience firsthand the "brutality" of men and their sexual desires. Ironically, much of the marital therapy advice at that time emphasized pleasure in marriage, and sexual fulfillment was viewed as essential for a "happy marriage." Women walked a thin line between sexual asceticism and nymphomania, and their pleasure was narrowly viewed as being at the hands of their skilled husbands. If a woman was never taught how to love, she was at risk of frigidity, which was defined as failing to reach vaginal orgasm or exhibiting lack of sexual desire. Hysteria, defined as chronic nervous and mental illness, was commonly diagnosed in the late nineteenth century and was thought to result from any number of difficulties related to sexuality, such as low or high desire or painful sex. With guiding textbooks such as *Frigidity in women: Its characteristics and treatment* (1948) and *Frigidity in woman: in relation to her love life* (1943),* women's sexuality has had a long history of being contained, reframed, prodded, exposed, and pathologized. Nonetheless, Freud contributed to a much greater public and professional awareness of sexuality, which led a new generation of sex researchers and clinicians to employ better-defined techniques in sex therapy.

MASTERS AND JOHNSON
AND THE IMPORTANCE OF TOUCH

IN THE 1950S and 1960s, William Masters and Virginia Johnson ushered in an entirely new era of behavioral sex therapy practices that challenged some of the tenets of traditional

---

* See Peter Cryle's 2009 article "A terrible ordeal from every point of view": (Not) managing female sexuality on the wedding night. Journal of the History of Sexuality, 18(1), 44-64 for more on this.

psychoanalysis. Sex therapy was brief, focused on a specific problem, and involved a therapist providing specific instructions on skills to practice. Masters, an obstetrician-gynecologist, and Johnson, a research associate and Masters's professional as well as personal partner, saw evidence of chronic stress and anxiety in many of their patients who complained of sexual dysfunction, and this paved the way for them to develop sensate focus therapy, which involved a series of structured touching exercises between two partners.

After observing hundreds of women (and men) engage in sexual activity in their research laboratory while their body responses were monitored with various pieces of psychophysiological machinery, Masters and Johnson postulated that anxiety was at the root of most sexual dysfunctions. They coined the term "spectatoring," in which a person watches themself vigilantly during sex and judges their own as well as their partner's performance instead of immersing themselves in the encounter. Spectatoring is associated with anxiety, negative judgment, and worries about a partner's thoughts and behaviors.

If you have ever found yourself focusing on whether you are responding in an "acceptable" way during a sexual encounter (note that only you are defining what is acceptable versus unacceptable), then you have experienced spectatoring. Masters and Johnson reasoned that spectatoring during sex elicits changes in the nervous system that block a person from fully immersing themself in the encounter and that the accompanying muscle tension and distraction prevents arousal and orgasm. As an antidote to spectatoring, Masters and Johnson reasoned that systematic touching between partners, with the goal of reducing anxiety and without the goal of triggering sexual arousal, is necessary to overcome this difficulty.

As a species, we respond automatically to touch. Emotions such as empathy or concern lead us to reach out to give someone a hug. Emotions can, however, also trigger the opposite effect—pushing someone away or retracting our own body in a reflexive manner. Couples in a new relationship delight in being in constant physical contact. Hand holding, kissing, and caressing are at their peak frequency in the first few months of a relationship but precipitously decline after that. Research presented in the 2012 book *The Normal Bar* on ninety thousand men and women around the world indicates that couples in a long-term relationship miss nonsexual touching and physical affection even more than they miss any decline in sexual frequency.

Sensate focus puts people back into physical contact with one another, without any specific goals related to sex. It involves a structured series of touching exercises in which the giver of the touch uses their own curiosity to touch all parts of the other partner's body in a nonsexual and nongoal-oriented way.* The touch is not meant to elicit sexual pleasure or orgasm. Instead, the giver of the touch is instructed to set aside their pre-existing beliefs about how a partner liked or wanted to be touched and instead to touch as if they were exploring that person's body for the first time. Think of your own relationships and whether you remember a period of total exploration in the early stages, where you could spend hours just touching each other. Like John Mayer's song "Your Body Is a Wonderland," which describes spending an afternoon discovering one another's bodies, this type of unbridled curiosity is what

---

* *For the interested reader, I recommend Linda Weiner and Constance Avery-Clark's 2017 book* Sensate focus in sex therapy: The illustrated manual. *New York: Routledge.*

sensate focus attempts to elicit. The receiver of the touch is instructed to notice the sensations without judgment.

Since couples are given strict instructions to abstain from sexual activity while practicing sensate focus, ideally, concerns about performance and the partner's expectations or disappointments typically associated with sex are eliminated. Even if one partner becomes sexually aroused while receiving touch, they are advised to notice the sensations in their body but to resist acting on any sexual feelings. They should not request sexual intercourse simply because they are aroused. (Of course, that can be easier stated than done.)

During the era of Masters and Johnson's pioneering work, couples would retreat to a clinic-hotel for a few weeks and practice sensate focus for several hours a day without the distractions of their daily lives. Participants' responses to the program were extremely positive, with up to 98 percent showing an improvement in their sexual functioning afterward. Nearly every person participating in Masters and Johnson's structured and intensive behavioral program benefited, and most of them had continued to experience satisfying sexual encounters when they were assessed five years later. No research team has ever been able to replicate those remarkable outcomes with any type of sex therapy intervention since, though admittedly, contemporary life also makes it impossible to steal away to a hotel for two or three weeks and abandon all of life's other demands while you touch your partner for several hours a day. Perhaps this type of retreat alone contributed as much to patients' gains as the therapy itself.

Other factors unique to Masters and Johnson's participants may also have contributed to the remarkable success of sensate focus: both the patients and the providers were highly motivated, and patients could afford the treatment. We know that a patient's commitment to therapy, regardless of the type of therapy that is being delivered, is one of the most important ingredients in a successful outcome. Moreover, patients who can afford sex therapy may be qualitatively different in some of the social determinants that directly affect sexual functioning. Not all individuals who struggle with a sexual concern have the means to pay for a private sex therapist. This calls into question how representative Masters and Johnson's patients were of the larger population of people who experience sexual dysfunction.

For a long time, sensate focus and, more generally, sex therapy practices that emphasized sexual pleasure and touching remained the mainstay of treatment for sexual dysfunction, and they continue to be widely used to this day. In their recent book, *Sensate Focus in Sex Therapy: The Illustrated Manual* (2017), Linda Weiner and Constance Avery-Clark refresh sensate focus therapy for the modern era and assist health-care providers in instructing their patients on the power and promise of sensate focus. Mutual pleasure in the absence of anxiety is the hallmark of this approach, which some experts view as foundational for sexual satisfaction in women as well as men.

Joanna's sex therapist used this brief, skills-based approach to guide some of her treatment, and Joanna benefited greatly from learning about the various reasons people have for engaging in sex. Also, in contrast to the psychoanalytic approach of the early twentieth century, where therapy may have continued for many years, these newer behavior-based therapies were much briefer and more structured, and rather than dredging through a person's childhood, they were focused on the specific sexual concern. Joanna's sex therapy consisted of approximately twelve sessions over the course of a year. She learned sensate focus and began to practice it weekly with her husband. Over time, the touching exercises taught Joanna to notice (for the first time) her own sexual sensations as her husband touched her. She was also challenged to hold back on her tendency to rush into intercourse (stemming from her belief that her husband *needed* intercourse), and she started to take pleasure in just being touched without any expectation of sex. She also felt increasingly comfortable providing her husband with feedback about which touches she liked—both their location and their intensity.

MEDICAL APPROACHES TO LOW DESIRE

THE SEXUAL REVOLUTION of the 1960s to 1970s was a period in which social norms regarding sexuality were challenged, and there was a general acceptance of sex outside of marriage. This was also a period of great medical advances, such as the birth control pill, and the legalization of abortion, which accompanied the rising role of women in society and feminism. The personal massager, or vibrator, which was invented in the late 1800s to treat hysteria in women by inducing paroxysms of the pelvic floor, was reclaimed by feminists during the sexual revolution for the sole purpose of inciting sexual pleasure. *Liberating Masturbation: A Meditation on Self Love*, by famed sexologist and artist Betty Dodson, was published in 1974. Dodson also led workshops for groups of women in New York City, teaching them to masturbate using vibrators. Cultural discourses on sex and pleasure were common, and some see this era as a high point in the history of women's sexuality. On the heels of the sexual revolution came a period of immense advances in sex therapy. Throughout the 1970s and 1980s, sex therapy programs emerged around the United States and the training of new sex therapists proliferated.

By the late 1980s and 1990s the tide had turned, and approaches to treating sexual problems took on a more medical focus as urology replaced psychiatry, psychology, and gynecology as a way of dealing with those problems. Important advances in the surgical treatment of erection problems as well as the discovery of a safe and effective injection therapy for erectile dysfunction meant that there was intense interest in the medical and biological causes of sexual problems. Even though sexual dysfunction was known to affect psychological experiences such as mood, anxiety, and personal well-being, the medical model dominated and pushed psychotherapy to the sidelines. With the approval of Viagra (sildenafil citrate) for the treatment of erectile dysfunction in the United States in 1998—and elsewhere around the world soon after that—there was now an alternative to penile injections that was discreet, effective, and relatively safe, and pharmaceutical companies quickly began to develop other medications aimed at restoring physical sexual response.

Throughout the 1990s there was exponential growth in the amount of research aimed at understanding the biological underpinnings of sexual arousal. Viagra and the erection problems it treated were no longer a private matter discussed behind closed doors. Public figures, such as former Senator Robert Dole, spoke publicly about erectile dysfunction, and Viagra prescriptions were in such high demand that physicians had to keep pre-printed prescription pads at their desks to keep up with the revolving door of new referrals. In 2000, 90 percent of men seeking treatment for erection problems received a prescription for either Viagra or one of the similarly acting medications (Levitra or Cialis). With the blockbuster success in pharmacologically enhancing men's sexual response, the obvious question was "What about women?"

Along with an explosion of interest in pharmacological treatments for sexual dysfunction, the first ever society strictly devoted to the study of women's sexual health was founded. Originally called the Female Sexual Function Forum (FSFF), it eventually became known as the International Society for the Study of Women's Sexual Health (ISSWSH). Some believed it was a platform for much of the pharmaceutical research into medications for women's sexual dysfunction, given that the annual meetings attracted much international interest from sexual medicine experts. Indeed, the society was dominated by medicine, and urology in particular. Before long, the medications that had restored men's erections were being tested in women with sexual difficulties. After all, given their epic success with men, wouldn't they be at least marginally helpful for women? However, they seemed to fall flat, barely increasing sexual desire and arousal scores compared with a placebo pill, and after millions of dollars had been spent by Viagra's sponsor, Pfizer Pharmaceuticals, in clinical trials with women, the company announced that it would no longer fund these trials. While Viagra did increase blood flow to the pelvic regions of the women participating in the clinical trials, it did nothing to improve their flat libido. But this was certainly not the end of the quest for the "pink Viagra" and, if anything, Viagra's failure intensified the race to be the first to find a drug to enhance female desire.

Procter & Gamble took a different approach—they developed a patch that delivered testosterone, through the skin, to women. For decades, it was believed that testosterone was the driver of women's (and men's) sexual desire. Indirect evidence for this came from studies showing that testosterone peaked at ovulation (when women are most fertile) and that this was also when women reported higher levels of sexual desire than during other phases of their menstrual cycle. Evolutionary psychologists explained this association by noting that the mid-cycle peak in testosterone would lead women to have more sex at a time when they were most fertile. Although many other studies failed to find a relationship between ovulation and sexual desire, and feminists regarded the pharmaceutical approach to studying women's sexual desire as marketing, the idea that testosterone was the driver of desire persisted.

In men, extremely low levels of testosterone—as in hypogonadism, a medical condition characterized by low testosterone, muscle weakness, and fatigue—lead to a total blunting of interest in sex, which treatment with testosterone seems to reverse. A large number of elegant scientific studies in which testosterone was given to women, either in pill form or via a patch placed on their skin, found that the hormone certainly increased women's sexual desire. But it also had many untoward side effects, such as acne and deepening of the voice, and there were concerns about the potential for testosterone to induce metabolic syndrome, a constellation of symptoms including high blood glucose levels, high triglyceride levels, low levels of HDL ("good" cholesterol), and high blood pressure, which collectively put a person at risk for cardiovascular disease. Some research also found that women who received testosterone may have had a greater risk of developing breast cancer than those in the placebo group. Promoters of the hormone challenged the science, noting that these women may have entered the clinical trial already at higher risk of breast cancer and that one could not conclude that their cancer was due to the testosterone treatment itself. To definitively make this connection, the study would have had to follow the women for years before and after their cancer developed.

Intrinsa was eventually approved in Europe for the treatment of "hypoactive sexual desire disorder" in postmenopausal women, though sales for the patch were not as robust as expected, and the buzz leading up to the approval of the patch in Europe seems to have fizzled. Hypoactive sexual desire disorder was a diagnosis defined by low or absent sexual desire and sexual fantasies, and an accompanying sense of significant distress. In North America at time of writing, testosterone is not approved for the treatment of low sexual desire in women, though some doctors do prescribe it "off label" after careful consideration of the risks versus benefits for each individual patient. But some women who are distressed by their low sexual desire are willing to try testosterone despite its off-label status in hopes of stirring up an inkling of sexual motivation.

In Joanna's situation, it is unlikely that the testosterone patch would have helped her much. In the clinical trials, testosterone was found to improve women's sexual desire, but it did little to improve their sexual satisfaction or feelings of pleasure. Nor did it affect women's beliefs about sexuality by, for example, empowering women to learn the triggers of their sexual arousal by giving them permission to explore their own bodies and to ask their partners for the kind of touch and stimulation they wanted. Nonetheless, many women and their partners ask for testosterone because it is far easier to slap on a hormone patch or slather on a cream than it is to reflect on what triggers or inhibits sexual response or to do exercises designed to overcome anxiety and low sexual self-esteem.

Joanna may have been tempted to ask her family physician to test her blood levels of testosterone. If that test had been done, it is most likely, however, that her testosterone levels would not have differed from those of women who were perfectly happy with their level of sexual desire.

Testosterone levels decline gradually throughout a woman's life until the menopause, when they reach about half the level they were when she was in her twenties. Population-based studies have found that women's sexual desire also declines with age, and it seemed reasonable to assume that these two processes were related—that the decline in sexual desire as a woman ages is due to a decline in her blood levels of testosterone. However, carefully conducted research that examined blood levels of testosterone in women with abundant levels of sexual desire and in women with distressing low sexual desire failed to find any significant difference in testosterone levels between the two groups. These findings led scientists to conclude that even if testosterone plays a role in women's loss of sexual desire, that role is likely small compared with the other factors contributing to her loss of desire. In other words, mood, sense of well-being, body image, self-esteem, and how a woman feels about her partner turned out to be far stronger predictors of her level of sexual desire than a single hormone.

We now know much more about the role of the brain in sex thanks to advances in neuroscience and neuroimaging. Studies comparing brain scans of women with healthy levels of sexual desire with those of women with low desire show differences in areas of the brain associated with motivation and in the encoding and retrieval of past experiences. Some experts interpret these findings as suggesting that women with low desire may spend more time monitoring and evaluating their own responses as opposed to attending to the erotic aspects of sexual cues. (This is explained in much more detail in Chapter 5.)

Other brain-imaging studies find that women with low desire have smaller areas of gray matter in the brain, and this may lead to decreased perception of sexual responses in the body. It is as if a barrier exists between a sexual trigger and the woman's response so that she does not register the trigger as sexual in the way that she may have in the past. As you might imagine, this may lead to significant frustration for the woman and her partner when what she used to find sexually arousing no longer elicits that same feeling of sexual motivation. It is as if her sexual radar has been turned off.

As scientists continue to be intrigued by the differences in brain structure and function between women who experience low sexual desire and those who do not, drug companies have focused their research on drugs to increase desire that target the brain. Many such drugs have been developed and tested, but as of 2017 the only one to win the race is flibanserin (trade name Addyi), originally made by Boehringer Ingelheim and then sold to Sprout Pharmaceuticals, which was bought by Valeant Pharmaceuticals in the summer of 2015, just two days after the Food and Drug Administration (FDA) announced the approval of Addyi for the treatment of hypoactive sexual desire disorder in women. Addyi was originally developed as an antidepressant medication, but when it was found to improve sexual desire more than patients' mood, Boehringer Ingelheim decided to develop a program of research evaluating Addyi as a drug to incite desire. Their sexual desire program was later continued by Sprout Pharmaceuticals, who took the Phase 3 clinical trials to the eventual FDA approval.

It was a long road to get to FDA approval, but Sprout Pharmaceuticals persisted in its efforts; the regulatory agency rejected the application twice before it finally approved it in August 2015. Over eleven thousand women with low desire participated in clinical trials in which they received Addyi and recorded their daily sex-related thoughts, behaviors, and satisfaction. Women receiving Addyi had one additional sexual encounter per month that they described as being satisfying to them than women receiving a placebo. Addyi did not lead the women to have more sex, however, and in fact, women participating in the clinical trials were already having sex, on average, about three times a month. This was a far cry from the experiences of Shelina, Susan, Cynthia, and Joanna, who were having sex only a few times a year.

It is on this last point that many experts have criticized Addyi and the drug company that makes and promotes it. Most of the women I see in my office are having enjoyable sex only a few times a year and would be elated to have rewarding sex a few times a month. Thus, it seems that the women who participated in the clinical trials leading to the approval of Addyi may be quite different from many, or perhaps even most, women who experience low sexual desire. Furthermore, the women participating in the Addyi studies had to meet very strict criteria to participate in one of the pivotal clinical trials. Specifically, they had to have reported losing the sexual desire that they once had and being distressed that, whereas they used to crave sex with their partners, now they did not think about it at all. They were still having sex a few times a month, but out of a sense of obligation rather than because they wanted sex for their own personal reward. The women in the studies also liked their partners; they had high levels of satisfaction with their relationship, were not depressed, were mostly physically healthy, and were not on any medications that might have interfered with sexual desire. In other words, the group of women who responded positively to Addyi were healthy, in happy relationships, and having relatively frequent sex, but they were just not feeling "horny," as they once did. If your own experience is quite different from that of the women in these studies, you might understandably feel skeptical that this medication would be useful for you.

What is particularly interesting to me, as a sex researcher and therapist, is that we really do not fully understand *how* Addyi works to improve (some) women's sexual desire. In studies carried out on rodents, Addyi was found to increase activity of the neurotransmitter dopamine and to decrease activity of the inhibitory brain chemical serotonin. It has been suggested that striking a balance between these two neurotransmitter systems improves women's sexual desire. Unfortunately, despite what drug promoters say, there have been no studies that show definitively that women have low sexual desire because their dopamine and serotonin systems are out of alignment. Furthermore, Addyi must be consumed daily, and research shows that benefits to sexual desire can only start to be seen after at least a month of use. Because of its side effects, such as dizziness and drops in blood pressure, and the strict recommendation that it not be mixed with alcohol, there has not been high demand for it. It is too early to tell whether Addyi will have a major effect on the large number of women who have low or no sexual desire, but if the number of prescriptions written in the first few weeks of Addyi's approval are any indication, it is not the blockbuster drug that many anticipated it would be. A mere two hundred or so prescriptions for Addyi were written in the first two weeks following its approval, compared with nearly half a million prescriptions of Viagra for men in the same span of time.

Will Addyi reverse Cynthia's deep sense of loss and regret about leaving her rewarding job so abruptly? Will tweaking Joanna's serotonin and dopamine levels inspire her to find her own voice and ask for what she wants sexually? Will the drug help restore some women's desire for sex in the face of ongoing and distressing genital pain? The answer to each of these questions is "likely not." In our culture of quick fixes, a pill has obvious appeal. But I do not believe that drugs to increase physiological responses, which many of the drugs before Addyi were, are the answer. Countless other women who participate in obligatory sex or sex with the sole intention of keeping a partner happy have only a distant memory of their own pleasure. Their motivation for sex may be low in part because the sex they have is not worth having. Many women with low sexual desire may not be experiencing a satisfying level of sexual arousal, and many may have never experienced an orgasm. Layered on top of these situations is unabated avoidance. Women with low sexual desire often avoid overt sexual encounters and even situations with the potential to lead to sex, such as going to bed at the same time as their partner. They may undress behind closed doors to avoid "turning a partner on," and some even deliberately start a fight at bedtime to kill a partner's sexual appetite.

Does this mean that women like Joanna are destined to live out the rest of their relationships engaging in sex without desire or, like millions of women, in a sexless relationship? The answer is no. Is medication likely to restore Joanna's lost sexual desire? In my opinion, the answer to this is also no. I have yet to be impressed by the lasting effects of such medications, and I believe that unless habitual patterns of avoidance, anxiety, catastrophic thinking, and negative self-judgment are changed, women will remain locked in their current unsatisfying experiences while being judgmental of themselves and their partners. Furthermore, the grip of stress and our penchant for multitasking are unlikely to be negated by a medication.

GETTING A HANDLE ON STRESS

FOR MANY WOMEN, managing stress is key to improving their sexual desire. Myriad studies have shown the strong link between chronic stress and sexual dysfunction in women, and stress can interfere with both emotional functioning and also thought patterns to decrease a woman's motivation for sex. In severe forms, stress can manifest as post-traumatic stress disorder (PTSD), which is diagnosed when someone has experienced or witnessed a significant traumatic event or accident and subsequently experiences chronic nightmares, hypervigilance (or being easily startled), or anxiety and re-experiences the traumatic event in their mind. Exposure to trauma can profoundly rupture an individual's sense of safety, sense of control in their world, and ability to trust and feel connected to others, features considered fundamental to healthy sexual functioning. In cases of chronic stress, it is possible that instead of triggering a sexual response, the early signs of sexual arousal trigger an alarm response or aggressive or fearful emotions.

Countless studies have shown that stress-reduction strategies, such as deep breathing (from the diaphragm) and progressive muscle relaxation, which have been in existence for nearly a hundred years, reduce feelings such as fear, anxiety, overwhelm, paralysis, hopelessness, and helplessness. These strategies also target negative thoughts associated with stress, such as "I am afraid that I will not be able to cope in this situation" and "I fear that my partner will leave me unless I have a good sexual response." They are especially effective at targeting the body's responses to a stressor, such as muscle tension, shortness of breath, and clammy hands.

Most stress-reduction strategies focus on eliciting the relaxation response, which is central to interrupting the stress cycle. In general, stress-reduction strategies can be grouped into behavioral techniques, such as relaxation, and cognitive techniques, such as cognitive challenging. We know that people can deliberately alter muscle tension by focusing on a particular area and intentionally either contracting (tightening) or relaxing (loosening) a muscle group. Moreover, there is evidence that if this type of deliberate relaxation is induced early enough in a stress response, it may effectively reduce the full-blown stress response. Cognitive challenging, on the other hand, involves identifying irrational thought patterns, challenging such thoughts, and then replacing them with more rational ways of thinking. When behavioral and cognitive strategies are combined, the resulting treatment is known as cognitive behavioral therapy (CBT).

Have you ever paid attention to your breathing when you were in a state of extreme stress? Chances are that you were breathing more quickly and shallowly, and that your breathing may have generated from your chest instead of your diaphragm. When you breathe from your chest, and not from your belly, you do not exhale enough carbon dioxide (the gas you produce when you breathe out), and the buildup of this gas can contribute to your feeling light-headed or nauseous.

Progressive muscle relaxation, perhaps the best-studied of the various relaxation techniques, involves progressively tightening and then relaxing each muscle group. The rationale behind first tensing the muscle can be understood by envisioning a pendulum. What happens when you pull the ball of the pendulum far over to the right and then let it go? The ball swings more swiftly through the center and over to the left. If you first tense a muscle group, the quality of the relaxation that follows the tension will be much deeper. In progressive muscle relaxation, you are guided to work on one muscle group at a time, first tensing it for about twenty seconds and then relaxing it for about forty seconds. A full progressive muscle relaxation exercise takes approximately twenty minutes to complete.

The technique known as cognitive challenging, which is a hallmark of CBT, involves challenging beliefs that may trigger anxiety or that may result from feeling chronically stressed. CBT consists of a structured set of steps in which you are first encouraged to identify beliefs or thoughts that are associated with anxiety. When you are feeling stressed or anxious, you may have a whole constellation of anxiety-related thoughts. Step 1 is to focus on one particular thought, such as "I fear that my partner will leave me unless I have a good sexual response." In Step 2, you are asked to analyze the validity of that thought by considering such factors as whether it is true, how logical it is, and what the probability is for it to be true. In this step, you also consider the evidence supporting the thought. In Step 3, you would examine counter-evidence to the thought by asking yourself the following questions:

1. Is there another way of looking at this thought?
2. Is there another explanation?
3. How would someone else consider the same situation?
4. Are my beliefs based on my emotions rather than on facts?
5. Am I setting unrealistic or unachievable standards for myself?
6. Am I forgetting relevant facts or overemphasizing other ones?
7. Am I engaging in all-or-nothing thinking?

Once you consider the evidence for the particular thought and the evidence against (with the against evidence far outweighing the for evidence in most cases), you then come up with a thought that is a more accurate reflection of reality and probabilities. This new belief will replace the original maladaptive belief you had.

Both the behavioral strategies and the cognitive strategies have been applied to improving sexual functioning in women (and men). In a review of all studies evaluating CBT for women with low sexual desire, CBT techniques are found to produce significant improvements in sexual desire, and a year following treatment, one-third of the women considered themselves to be completely symptom-free. Furthermore, many of the specific dysfunctional beliefs associated with sexual dysfunction (for example, my partner will leave me; I am sexually broken; my body does not become aroused) changed with treatment, and the women's partners expressed fewer unrealistic expectations and showed less rigidity in sex roles, a more positive attitude toward sexuality, and fewer doubts about themselves and their partner. The women also showed far fewer "musts" and "shoulds" in their thinking patterns.

Although one-third of the women were completely symptom-free after adopting these strategies, two-thirds continued to experience symptoms of low sexual desire after treatment. The authors of the study acknowledge that other strategies may be necessary to amplify the reductions in stress and improvements in women's sexual desire and sexual satisfaction. For women like Cynthia and Joanna, progressive muscle relaxation and cognitive challenging might have been sufficient to improve their anxiety so that they could feel less stress in their day-to-day lives. It might have been sufficient for improving their sexual desire also, translating into real and lasting improvements in their sexual relationships. For some women, however, a different approach is needed—one that entails a more fundamental change in how they live their lives. The strategies involve altering aspects of their body's and mind's reactions. In other words, we can teach the mind to have a more measured, and less reactive, response to stressful situations, and the body to respond to stress with less muscular tension and a higher tolerance level for stress.

But what if you could experience lasting improvements in stress, anxiety (including panic attacks), sexual desire, and overall quality of life by not changing? What? Not changing? This seems entirely paradoxical, and yet, it is the crux of mindfulness meditation techniques. Mindfulness is about fully inhabiting the present moment, without trying to change anything. It involves a complete acceptance of who you are and what your experience is—without judgment. Could it be that in our efforts to change our sexuality, to reach some idealized standard of what we are told is "normal" sexual desire, we generate stress that further impedes our true sexual potential? What if fully experiencing the present moment, including all of the ups and downs of emotions and thoughts, could lead to a satisfying sexual life without the grief of trying to change anything at all? Not only is mindfulness an important ingredient in disabling the vicious cycle of stress-anxiety-dysfunctional beliefs-sexual dysfunction, it is also a *crucial* ingredient in enabling women to cultivate sexual desire. I believe that stress management and learning to live in the present moment are key to cultivating sexual desire. Mindfulness meditation, which has been found to consistently and robustly reduce stress, may be the single most effective way of attaining sexual satisfaction.

CHAPTER 3

INTRODUCING THE RAISIN

The best cure for the body is a quiet mind.

NAPOLÉON BONAPARTE

S ARAH IS A thirty-two-year-old college instructor living
with her fiancé, Seojun, a senior executive for a mining
company. In the first few weeks after they met, Sarah
and Seojun had many adventures and exciting experiences.
They took spontaneous weekend trips to charming destina-
tions, dined at the best restaurants in town, and danced until
dawn and until their feet ached. Their sex was fiery and frequent, and they felt an ease with one another that they had
not experienced with past partners. They experimented with
role playing during sex, in which each would take on a different character to enact their fantasies. Sarah enjoyed taking on
a dominant role and would give strict commands to Seojun
about how she wanted to be pleased sexually. She took pleasure in aggressive sex and occasionally blindfolded Seojun,
whose feelings of surprise and anticipation further contributed to the heat of their sexual encounters. Seojun readily took

on the submissive role, finding it a welcome reprieve from his job, where he continually provided direction and leadership to his staff of nearly a hundred.

At first Sarah was very satisfied with her level of sexual desire and with the sex she and Seojun were having. But about six months into the relationship, her level of desire began to wane, as it had done in each of her previous three long-term relationships. She recognized the pattern: as she became more attached to Seojun, sex became more routine, less experimental, and less exciting. One evening while having sex with Seojun, Sarah caught herself making a grocery list in her mind and realized that she had slipped far away from the invigorating and electrifying sexual experiences she used to have. Her feelings of passion began to fade, and she felt less motivation to have sex with Seojun. As a result, the sex they were having became less satisfying. She certainly did not crave it in the way she had when they first met. Typically, Sarah would break up with a partner when her desire began to dwindle. With Seojun, however, things were different. She loved him, as well as the sex they had, and she did not want her relationship with him to end, as she envisioned a long future with him. At the same time, she worried that her lost desire was a symptom that this relationship was "not meant to be." Sarah had always believed that when she found "the one," her passion for sex would endure.

Sarah had experienced anxiety throughout her lifetime. She described herself as a perfectionist who strove to excel in all her activities. She was class valedictorian during her senior year of high school, was chosen as chair of the board for her housing complex, and volunteered on several committees in the college where she worked. Her job as a college instructor was rewarding, and she poured an immense amount of time into perfecting every lecture. Her relationship with the students in her classes was of utmost importance to her, and she would be distraught whenever she received a poor evaluation from a student in her class, even if most of the evaluations were good.

Sarah's anxiety was centered on fear of failure. She imagined catastrophic outcomes and expected that others would ridicule her as a result. This anxiety kept her focused on monitoring others' behavior toward her. She was hyper-attuned to signs in other people, such as a furrowed brow, which she interpreted as a sign of disapproval. She obsessed about whether her coworkers admired her, though she firmly believed that they looked down on her. Although Sarah did not have panic attacks, she frequently experienced tightness in her neck and shoulders, a rapid heart rate, and quickened chest breathing, especially during times of high stress, such as before deadlines or before her annual performance review.

Sarah's life was immensely busy, but she believed she was skilled at multitasking and able to keep all of her balls in the air. She thrived on being busy, and when asked what emotion she liked the least, she responded, "Being bored."

As sex with Seojun became less novel and therefore less exciting, Sarah's mind began to wander. At first she didn't notice that she was thinking about other, nonsexual matters. She trusted that her body "knew what to do" and that it would respond automatically to Seojun's touch. About a year into the relationship, when it started taking longer and longer for her to reach orgasm, she blamed stress at work for the problem. She was teaching two new courses that she had designed, and she felt that her students and faculty coworkers would be scrutinizing the course material. She experienced the occasional panic attack during that six-month period, but when the courses proved to be a great success, her anxiety returned to its typical low-to-moderate level. However, the quality of her orgasms did not return. They continued to feel like a dull blip on the screen, without the feelings of euphoria that she recalled from the past.

Sarah and Seojun had been engaged for three years, but at Sarah's request they delayed setting a date for their wedding pending an improvement in their sex life. She loved Seojun deeply and was wholly committed to him, but she believed her low level of desire for sex needed to be resolved before she could marry him. She was increasingly preoccupied with the belief that Seojun may not be "the one" given the fizzle of her spark for him, and this thought led to great distress for her. It was at that point that Sarah contacted me for sex therapy.

Sarah's loss of sexual desire may be related to several factors. Anxiety is associated with low sexual desire, and we know that daily stress interferes with sexual response. Sarah was afraid of performance failure, and she was a perfectionist, leading her to scrutinize the sex she and Seojun were having and to judge each encounter as either "good" or "bad." She was a spectator of the encounter rather than an active and engaged participant. And as she slipped into watching more than participating, her body's sexual response was further blunted and she desired sex even less.

Sarah's tendency to try to multitask also likely played a key role in her poor sexual response. Because she believed that sex was like a reflex, and that she should experience an automatic sexual response to Seojun's touch, she started to put less effort into sex, and her mind would wander. She would get lost in myriad thoughts that had nothing to do with the sexual encounter. Her delayed and muted orgasms, and eventual failure to have an orgasm, were a direct result of insufficient sexual arousal because she was disengaged. Her body was going through the sexual motions, but her mind was elsewhere. As her sexual arousal lessened, sex became less satisfying, and her motivation for this mediocre sex understandably declined in a parallel manner.

As I described these possible contributors to Sarah after she shared her story with me, she fully agreed with my analysis and in particular with my suggestion that her mind had become disengaged from the sexual interaction and that, as a result, her body had started to respond less to sexual triggers. Even though the activities she and Seojun engaged in would at one time have elicited positive sexual feelings, her preoccupied mind meant that those triggers were muted. We reasoned that if she worked on bringing her mind back to the sexual encounter, she might start to regain pleasurable sexual feelings, and over time, her motivation for this more satisfying sex would increase. I explained that her mind was trained to multitask, and that retraining it to remain in the present would take concerted effort.

THE GAS AND BRAKE PEDALS OF SEX

PERHAPS YOU CAN relate to Sarah's experience. I hear similar complaints all too often in my clinical practice: my body responds, but my mind is preoccupied. A drug like Viagra, designed to improve genital blood flow, would do little to re-engage Sarah's mind and might result in additional frustration that the "treatment" did little to increase her desire from apathetic to ignited. Research on the factors associated with sexual desire shows that it can be helpful to think about two categories of factors: the facilitators (which researchers refer to as excitation) and the inhibitors (which researchers refer to as inhibition). Together these factors form the dual control model of sexual response. Facilitators include the woman's level of arousability, scents, power dynamics between her and a partner, and aspects of the environment, such as the calming flicker of a candle or the mellow sounds of jazz music. Inhibitors of sexual response include being easily distracted while sexually aroused, being concerned about sexual performance, and needing things to be "just right" in order to feel sexually in the mood.

Many treatments focus on attempts to increase the facilitators of sexual response, such as applying a stronger sexual stimulus, encouraging women to apply more lubricants, or using off-label medications that increase genital blood flow. However, research suggests that inhibition may be a more important factor in women's low desire than the lack of facilitators or excitation. In her book *Come as You Are*, Emily Nagoski uses the analogy of the gas and brake pedals of a car to illustrate this. She argues that many of our approaches to sex therapy have missed the mark by focusing on ways to increase the pressure on the gas pedal (more excitation). She believes that we should focus instead on lessening the pressure placed on the brake pedal (less inhibition). When you consider your own sexual desire, is your gas pedal barely being tapped, or is your brake pedal being forced to the car floor? Considering whether you have too many inhibitors or not enough facilitators can help steer you toward the best treatment option.

A large body of research carried out at the Kinsey Institute in Bloomington, Indiana, has supported this dual control model of sexual response and shows that women need to identify and alter those inhibiting forces that buffer sexual desire and arousal. What's more, a woman's degree of sexual inhibition can predict her level of sexual desire not only in the present but also in the future. In other words, inhibitions can forecast a future of sexual problems down the road, so they are worth paying attention to. Sarah had a list of inhibitors hampering her sexual desire.

Sarah is an ideal candidate for the array of practices that make up mindfulness meditation, in which you meditate while focusing on either your breath or a particular part of your body. Here is how it works if you are focusing on your breath.

Noticing the Breath

1. Close your eyes and get into a comfortable position, taking notice of your posture and the points of contact between your body and your surroundings.
2. Gently move your attention toward the breath. This may include paying attention to each in-breath and each out-breath, as well as the types of sensations in your nostrils, your chest, and elsewhere.
3. As you continue to focus on the sensations associated with breathing, you may start to notice when the in-breath changes to the out-breath and when the out-breath circles around to the next in-breath. You may become quite skilled at deciphering all of the individual sensations associated with breathing, including the breath's rate, pace, depth, and location, as well as whether there are sounds associated with breathing, whether there is tension in the body, and whether you want to continue noticing your breath or you want to move away from noticing it.

During a typical mindfulness practice, whether you are paying attention to your breath or to a specific location in the body, your mind will remain present for a while but then will likely drift—to other physical locations in the body, to sounds inside the room or outside the window, and almost inevitably to thoughts such as "Am I doing this correctly?" "Is this relaxing me?" "Has it improved my sexual functioning yet?" "Why do I find this so difficult?" "I am not cut out to meditate." "How am I going to deal with this difficult situation with my boss?" "Are we out of milk?" And on and on. Mindfulness is not only about paying attention, it is also about *how* we pay attention—nonjudgmentally.

MILLENNIA OF MINDFULNESS

MINDFULNESS IS NOT a new practice; it has been in existence for close to four thousand years. Although it is commonly associated with Buddhism, there is evidence that mindfulness was practiced long before the Buddha formalized it as an element of Buddhism. As Bhikkhu Sujato summarizes in his book *A History of Mindfulness*, the term "mindfulness" was a translation of *sati*, which means memory and was used by the Brahmans to refer to the memorization of scriptures. Memorizing these vast texts required a mental state of clarity and focus that was free of distractions. Mindfulness practice was necessary for the development of insight, or an awareness of the true reality of things. Therefore, mindfulness cultivated a clarity of focus that allowed one to know truth.

There are two types of Buddhist mindfulness: Samatha and Vipassana. In Samatha meditation, the focus is mostly on concentration training and building the skill of sustained attention. For example, transcendental meditation is one type of concentration-based meditation approach. In Vipassana meditation, or insight training, meditators are aware of the objects in focus, but they also pay attention to the changing and unfolding of their experience, moment by moment. In Buddhism, mindfulness is considered to be an antidote to delusion and a prerequisite for the attainment of insight.

Although there has been some disagreement within the literature about the definition of mindfulness, it seems that many Buddhist teachers believe that it is a combination of nonjudgmental awareness of sensations in the here-and-now and the retention of that information. During mindfulness, the person who is meditating uses an anchor point, such as the breath, to focus their attention on the present moment and notices the quality of sensations that are associated with breathing, such as those that make up the entire in-breath and out-breath, the rate and sound of breathing, and the physical sensations at the chest and nostrils while the person is inhaling and exhaling. In signal-to-noise parlance, it is as if the signal strength has become so strong as a result of the concentration and the noise in the background has faded so much that one is able to focus on the signal for a very long period of time without being distracted.

Samatha training ends there, with a continual redirection of the person's attention to the breath the moment the mind loses focus and goes elsewhere. Vipassana training, however, adopts a much wider landscape of focus, so that the person who is meditating on the sensations of breathing may be aware of other sensations, sounds, and thoughts. Thus, they are aware that these other sensations, sounds, and thoughts have become the new focus of attention, but they still maintain an awareness of the sensations of breathing farther back in their field of awareness. They are continually aware of where their attention is, and with this practice they give themselves permission to be right where they are, even if they are not focusing on the original target. It is not about "turning off" other distractions but rather about accepting that myriad other sensations come into and out of a person's focus and that the person can attend to whichever aspect of the field they wish to. Such a dispassionate attitude toward intrusions into one's attention is thought to be important for helping one to stay with the current object of their attention without becoming distressed, judging themselves negatively, or thinking that they are simply not able to meditate.

In the mid-1970s, mindfulness started to make its way into mainstream Western medicine and society. Jon Kabat-Zinn is typically credited with catalyzing this transition, beginning when he was a postdoctoral fellow at MIT and attended a lecture by Philip Kapleau, a Zen Buddhist teacher. Transformed by what he heard, Kabat-Zinn started meditating that day and eventually gave up a career as a molecular biologist to study and teach meditation, putting it into a modern-day secular context and developing an eight-week program that guided participants through meditation practices and included a daily forty-five-minute at-home practice and a full-day mindfulness retreat. He focused on patients suffering from chronic intractable pains who, despite months and even years of trying to reduce their pain, did not benefit from the conventional medical and surgical treatments given to them at the pain clinic at the University of Massachusetts Medical Center. He told them that "as long as you are breathing, there is more right with you than there is wrong, no matter how ill or how hopeless you may feel,"* meaning that anyone with a pulse is equipped with all they need to be mindful.

---

* Jon Kabat-Zinn (1990). Full catastrophe living: Using the wisdom of your body and mind to face stress, pain, and illness. New York: Delacorte Press, p. 2.

Armed with little more than hope and an ability to gently guide patients' awareness to their breath and body, including the pains that made their lives barely livable, Kabat-Zinn put the Eastern Buddhist practice into a medical context and simplified the language to remove any religious references or undertones. He would guide a group of patients with "Pay attention to your breath. Notice the movement of your chest as the cool air comes in and the warm air leaves. Pay attention to the beginning of the in-breath, the middle of the in-breath, and the end of the in-breath. Now pay attention to the beginning, middle, and end of the out-breath." Over the course of a structured eight-week group treatment, Kabat-Zinn taught patients with diverse and debilitating chronic pain how to eat mindfully, to pay attention to their breath, to become aware of physical sensations in their bodies, and to treat thoughts simply as by-products of brain activity—something to be noticed but not to be swept away by.

He also discovered that his eight-week program led to striking improvements in patients' pain levels and quality of life. His work eventually paved the way for the development of a formalized program known as mindfulness-based stress reduction (MBSR) and the creation of the Center for Mindfulness in Boston at the University of Massachusetts.

As a scientist, Kabat-Zinn also studied the outcomes of his groups, measuring different aspects of patients' experiences, including pain intensity, mood, and quality of life before and after they participated in his eight-week program. He observed that several domains of physical and mental health not only improved but also remained improved long after the program had ended. People were getting back into their lives and learning to accept that chronic pain could come along for the ride. The publication of his *Full Catastrophe Living* in 1990—which described in detail how mindfulness was delivered to sufferers of chronic pain and shared the science behind improvements in pain intensity, stress, and quality of life—led many scientists and clinicians to turn to mindfulness as a possible treatment for other conditions and to a demand by health-care providers for instruction in how to deliver mindfulness to their own patients.

Over the next two decades, variations of mindfulness-based stress reduction were developed, including the extremely well studied and implemented mindfulness-based cognitive therapy (MBCT), which was developed to prevent the recurrence of a major depressive episode in people with a history of depression by teaching them to live fully in the moment and to notice when they might be starting to experience depressive symptoms. Mindfulness practices guided them to fully attend to their current feelings and thoughts and to curb the tendency to think in future-oriented ways such as, "Oh no! My depression is back! This means I will not be able to function in my relationships, in my job, and in my community." Such hopeless thoughts about the future are hallmark signs of a depressive episode. Mindfulness guides participants to remain in the present moment, to pay attention to sensations in the body, and to view catastrophic thoughts as passing events of the mind rather than truths to be attended to.

Rates of depressive relapse were 50 percent less likely after mindfulness training. Mindfulness-based cognitive therapy linked the mindfulness practices developed by Kabat-Zinn with cognitive therapy for depression and cognitive science on the purported mechanisms by which people experience a depressive relapse after a period of not having any symptoms of depression. The simple rationale for why people may have a depressive relapse is that during periods of distress, people resort to old patterns of depressive thinking and automatic thoughts, and the persistence of these thinking patterns can trigger another depressive episode.

Mindfulness is a way of relating to thoughts in an entirely different way. A thought can be viewed as a "mental sensation" in the same way that movements of the belly and chest are observed as "breath sensations." Mindfulness-based cognitive therapy encourages patients to observe thoughts as "passing events of the mind" rather than something that needs to be attended to or believed. So often when we have a troubling thought, it leads to another one, which in turn leads to another one, and before we know it, several minutes (or hours or weeks or even months) have elapsed. Guided meditations allow the participant to watch these thoughts, as if from a distance, without reacting emotionally to them. Acceptance of these thoughts is key; the participant practices observing thoughts in a nonjudgmental way and accepting whatever it is that arises. Because we have a tendency to judge ourselves and others in many domains of our lives, practicing acceptance and nonjudgment can be challenging. For some of us, letting go of our habitual tendency to judge can feel downright unattainable. (We will consider this mindfulness of thoughts practice in more detail in Chapter 5.)

With the explosion of interest in mindfulness-based stress reduction and mindfulness-based cognitive therapy, and with therapist training programs, institutes, and week-long retreats taking place all over the world, mindfulness has also been extended to people suffering from various psychological as well as physical ailments beyond chronic pain and depression. Mindfulness-based stress reduction is routinely offered to cancer patients undergoing treatment as a way of helping them to become active participants in their own treatment and care plans rather than passive recipients and bystanders. Elana Rosenbaum's 2005 book *Here for Now: Living Well with Cancer Through Mindfulness* details Rosenbaum's own experiences of practicing and teaching mindfulness during three cancer episodes. Her journey provides guidance for other survivors to follow.

During chemotherapy, the survivor may be guided to notice sensations of nausea—where they are, their intensity, and what individual sensations make up the larger, uncomfortable ones. During appointments with her oncologist, when a woman may be anxious and fearful, the survivor may be guided to notice sensations of breathing, and the array of mental events that present as worries, fears, and anger. Fatigue can also be observed with kindness and acceptance. Scientific evidence shows that mindfulness improves cancer survivors' ability to cope psychologically and improves physiological factors such as immune function and decreases cortisol—the stress hormone. People with cancer who participated in mindfulness-based stress reduction also showed improved tumor marker activity, similar to that of a cancer-free control group, indicating a slowdown in the progression of the cancer. Because of its positive effects on both the mind and the body, mindfulness is now offered, and even encouraged, in many major North American cancer centers.

Today, mindfulness is routinely offered to people struggling with fear, phobias, and panic attacks and has been found to help not only people in the throes of an anxiety attack, but also people in general to allow them to be more relaxed. Mindfulness has also been applied to behavioral problems in children, such as attention deficit/hyperactivity disorder, and has been adopted in many elementary schools as a part of the daily curriculum, where it has been found to increase children's own ratings of their happiness as well as their likability as rated by their peers. Dozens of books have been written for those with various health conditions, and for those who simply wish to be more present in their lives, on how to benefit from the power of the present moment with nonjudgmental awareness. Couldn't we all benefit from being a little less judgmental of others and of ourselves?

Moment by moment and breath by breath, these mindfulness programs have allowed thousands of people to be engaged more fully in their own lives and to benefit both emotionally and physically as a result. Mindfulness was featured on the front cover of the February 3, 2014, *Time* magazine with the heading "The Mindful Revolution." The accompanying article described it as anything but a fad. In fact, financial advisers in Silicon Valley; executives from Google, Twitter, and Facebook; congressmen; the U.S. Department of Defense; and countless institutes and corporations have set up programs and settings in which staff can practice mindfulness. It turns out that the daily practice of mindfulness can help employees perform better, buffer the effects of disruptions in the workplace on accuracy, improve communication, facilitate open listening, and cultivate better leadership qualities. Overall, it makes employees happier and more productive.

THE RAISIN

HOW COULD MINDFULNESS help with Sarah's low sexual desire? Because she spent little time attending to the present moment and instead was caught in a wave of thoughts and worries about the future, Sarah was an ideal candidate for learning mindfulness. Whether repeatedly reviewing past events or thinking about what might happen in the future, she was missing out on the here-and-now.

She enrolled in a mindfulness-based sex therapy program led by the Department of Obstetrics and Gynaecology at the University of British Columbia in collaboration with the British Columbia Centre for Sexual Medicine in Vancouver. Our team of mindfulness facilitators* created an eight-week program that was tested and refined over several years, then tested again. Many of the publications arising from this extensive body of research can be found at brottolab.com. We led these group sessions in board rooms located in a busy medical clinic and with a sign on their doors that read "Quiet please. Mindfulness taking place inside." Sarah and the seven other women in the group were introduced to mindfulness with a simple exercise. Each woman was given a raisin, along with the following instructions from the group facilitator.

1. Observe the object. We are going to refer to this as an object, even if you recognize this and immediately know the name of it. By calling it an object, we are encouraging you to encounter this object as if for the first time.
2. Take note of its shape, size, color, and contour.
3. Notice how the light reflects off its surface.
4. Smell the object, taking in the various aromas.

---

* During 2003–2016, as our various mindfulness-based groups were being developed, we had a large group of dedicated psychologists, psychiatrists, sexual medicine physicians, nurses, students, and mindfulness experts contribute to the program. I am indebted to the following individuals: Rosemary Basson, Andrea Grabovac, Mijal Luria, Kelly Smith, Miriam Driscoll, Monique Rees, Amy Wagner, Craig Sawchuk, Mark Lau, Marie Carlson, and Laurel Paterson, among others.

5. Notice how your body responds to those aromas.
6. Lift it to your ear.
7. If you move it between your fingers, does it have a sound?

There was a long pause between each instruction as the women lifted the raisin to their eyes, nose, and ears. The group facilitator continued, again with long pauses between the instructions.

8. Put the object against your lips without opening them.
9. Notice how it feels.
10. Notice if your mouth or body starts to react to having it there.

The group facilitators could hear the women salivating as they anticipated putting the raisin in their mouth.

11. Now put the object in your mouth and roll it around with your tongue. Try not to bite it. What sensations do you notice? This can be a sharp example of how your mind anticipates something, and reacts physiologically to it by preparing for it.

After another long pause, the facilitator continued.

12. Eventually put the object between your back teeth and slowly and deliberately take one bite. Notice the explosion of flavors. Can you decipher the different flavors? Can you observe where one flavor ends and the next one begins?

13. Then, very slowly chew into the object and follow the tra-. jectory of its contents as they move down your esophagus. Notice the aftertaste and the echo of the aftertaste.

During this introductory mindfulness exercise, which is somewhat standard across mindfulness-based group programs for other conditions, the women participating in our groups often report that the raisin looks like a vulva. When asked what they noticed as they looked at, touched, smelled, and tasted the raisin, most usually describe an array of different reactions to the raisin, describing in detail its valleys and ridges, commenting on how the light reflects off its surface, and stating that they had never noticed the part of the raisin that was previously the stem of a grape. They look awed as they detail its physical properties. Like the participants in other mindfulness-based cognitive therapy or mindfulness-based stress reduction groups, the women with sexual concerns participating in our group sessions remarked how tempting it was to chew the raisin as soon as the facilitator passed the plate around.

When asked how eating and interacting with the raisin in this way was different from how they normally ate raisins at home, most of the women in Sarah's group broke out into a gentle laugh. "I usually grab a big handful and throw them into my mouth, usually with a few missing the target and landing on the floor," one woman said. "I don't even think about them, I just eat," said another. Some commented on the reference to the raisin as an "object" rather than as "a raisin." "I suppose this is so that we approach it with fresh eyes," said one woman.

The facilitator then asked the women: "How is eating the raisin in this way relevant to the sexual desire concerns that brought you to this group?" After a very brief pause, one woman stated, "Like eating a handful of raisins, I just go through the motions during sex. I don't slow down to experience all of the different sensations of touch, sound, smell, taste even! I go on autopilot. My mind is thinking about other things, usually unrelated to sex. Maybe if I paid more attention during sex, like I did to the shape, color, and taste of this raisin, I'd realize that there were so many enjoyable aspects of sex that I don't pay attention to. Maybe paying attention is the key to unlocking my lost sexual desire."

As the women are asked about their observations during the mindful eating and how this practice might be relevant to their own sexuality, they immediately comprehend the power of mindfulness and its potential role in healing their sexual difficulties. We rarely provide this explanation to women before they take part in the mindfulness practice and prefer that they draw these conclusions independently.

Even after running dozens of groups with hundreds of women, I am always struck by how the women in these groups come to these observations so readily. I rarely, if ever, need to "sell" mindfulness to them. In this one exercise of paying attention to all aspects of their sensory experience while interacting with and eating one raisin, they feel alive, and they see this "aliveness" as being missing from sex.

Sarah's homework was to eat one meal a day mindfully. She was encouraged to put down her fork between bites and even close her eyes to fully take notice of the sensations and flavors in her mouth. It is a wonderful way to introduce group members to mindfulness because it powerfully illustrates our ability to move the focus of attention to a single object, and many people can relate to gobbling down a mouthful of food without giving it any thought. One of the two facilitators always guides the group mindfulness practices in-session. For the week between sessions, participants are given either written instructions for their daily practice or an audiorecording of the practice that they can use. Immediately after every in-session mindfulness practice, the facilitators guide the women through an "inquiry." Some mindfulness experts consider the inquiry to be the heart of a mindfulness practice.

The inquiry has three components, all intended to help a participant observe and reflect on what arises during the mindfulness practice. The facilitator asking questions during the three-part inquiry exhibits curiosity, compassion, and a deep sense of exploration when asking about a participant's experiences.

The first question facilitators ask women is "What did you notice and what sensations did you experience during this practice of observing the raisin?" Women will describe changes in their breathing rate and heart rate, that they notice changes in their muscle tension, or that they feel shifts in particular areas of pain in their body. We guide them to pay close attention to unfolding sensations, and they describe, in exquisite detail, aspects of their sensations and feelings that surprise even them: "I never knew that eating a single raisin could lead to so many different types of sensations!"

The second question is "How is this way of paying attention different from how you normally experience the day-to-day events of your life?" To this, women share that they typically knock back a handful of raisins, barely chewing, and then swallowing. Before the raisin remnants have made their way down the esophagus, the woman will report reaching for the next handful of raisins to swallow. Therefore, paying attention to the raisin in the way they did during this exercise is wildly different from how they normally pay attention to raisins, or food, in their lives.

In the third component of the inquiry, the facilitator asks about the relevance of the mindfulness practice they just did and the concerns about sexual desire they are struggling with. We ask, "How might paying attention to a raisin, as you did in this practice together, be useful or relevant to your current concerns about sexual desire?"

"Perhaps I need to slow down and savor the sex I am having, and that by rushing through it, I am missing so many exquisite details," one woman says. Another woman adds, "I realized that imagining swallowing the raisin was enough to make my mouth salivate. Maybe this is related to sex because I can think about a sexual scene and it can trigger arousal in my body." And another woman states, "There are many visual aspects of sex that I miss out on by keeping my eyes closed throughout. I realized that visual stimulation can be very powerful for making the experience more intense."

Whether you have never practiced mindfulness in your life or you have a regular meditation practice, I encourage you to try the following eating meditation now. You may choose to read through the following exercise in full before moving on to the practice. Alternatively, the Internet offers an assortment of free audioguides of the eating meditation, delivered in slightly different ways. For example, Bob Stahl has a YouTube video entitled "Raisin Meditation"* that you can use if you prefer to be guided through the instructions.

---

* See youtube.com/watch?v=tYDXQQBojk8

As you practice, it is likely that your mind will wander. This is not your fault, and it does not mean you are doing the exercise incorrectly. When this happens, you are encouraged to just notice this and gently bring your attention back to the raisin. There is as much mindfulness in noticing that your mind has wandered off somewhere away from the raisin as there is in continually paying attention to the raisin.

Eating Meditation: The Raisin

1. Start by examining the object.
2. Notice what details you can observe by looking at it.
3. Notice the color of the object, studying its texture.
4. Become aware of the details on the object's surface, patches of light and dark, reflections, and the sensation of it lightly resting on the palm of the hand.
5. Study the object intently.
6. Touch the object with a finger. Is it rough or smooth? Thick or thin? Hard or soft?
7. Notice the topography of the object. Look at the valleys and peaks.
8. Feel the weight of the object, and how it feels in the hand.
9. Pick the object up and touch it with a finger. Is it rough or smooth? Thick or thin? Hard or soft?
10. Lift the object to the nose and smell it. Observe the beginning, middle, and end of the aroma. Move the object to the other nostril and observe the aroma there.
11. Bring the object to one ear and roll it between the fingers. Notice any sounds.
12. Bring the object to the lips and rest it against the lips.

Let the lips feel what it feels like. Notice if your attention has moved to a thought about the object or anticipation of eating it. Allow this thought to be the new focus of attention until it fades away. Then return your attention to sensations in the body associated with the object.

13. Perhaps notice saliva building in the mouth. Bring a friendly interest to the various sensations as they arise, unfold, and fade away.

14. Place the object in the mouth, on the tongue, without chewing it.

15. Close the eyes and notice how it feels.

16. Focus on how it feels on the tongue.

17. Place the object between the teeth, without chewing it, and feel what it feels like between the teeth.

18. When you are ready, begin to chew the object slowly and thoroughly, focusing on its taste and texture.

19. Feel the teeth biting through the surface and taste the juice flowing over the tongue and mouth.

20. Notice the trajectory of the flavor as it bursts forth, the flood of saliva, how the flavor changes.

21. Notice the contraction of the muscles in the jaw when chewing.

22. When you're ready, swallow the object and observe the sensations of it passing down the throat.

23. Notice the sensations in the mouth, the taste and texture.

24. Whenever some other object, such as a physical sensation in another area of the body, a sound, or a thought becomes predominant, momentarily take this to be the new focus for attention and bring the same level of mindful awareness to that sensation, sound, or thought, continuing to observe it until it is no longer predominant. Then bring your attention back to the object.

25. And whenever you're ready, allow the eyes to open if they have been closed.

You can then move through the three levels of inquiry that were discussed earlier. First, what physical sensations did you notice? What other sensations were you aware of? Could you describe those sensations in even more detail? How long did those sensations last? How did you know the taste was sweet? What part of the tongue tasted sweetness? Did it stay the same over time or did it shift in any way? If so, in what way? Did you notice an impulse or urge to chew? If so, how did you first notice that impulse/urge? How did you become aware of it?

Next, consider how being aware of a raisin in this way is different from how you normally interact with (that is, consume) raisins. Specifically, how was paying attention to eating a raisin in this way different from how you might normally eat a raisin?

Finally, consider how this exercise might be relevant to your own experience of sexuality. If you experienced some salivation while the raisin was in your mouth before you began chewing, could this teach you anything about your own anticipation of sex? Do you anticipate certain outcomes of events before they even happen? Do you anticipate disastrous outcomes from sex with a partner, such as a lack of your own response or negativity from a partner's response? How might observing the link between expecting to chew the raisin and the mouth's salivation in anticipation of chewing be relevant to how you anticipate events in your own life?

HOW MUCH IMPROVEMENT IS THERE?

YOU MAY BE wondering how much of an improvement in their sexual desire women experience as a result of practicing mindfulness. In a typical scientific experiment of this type, women fill out validated self-report questionnaires before beginning the mindfulness group. They complete the same questionnaires again a few weeks after the eight-session mindfulness program has ended. We then use statistical tests to measure whether the change from pre- to post-mindfulness is statistically significant. When the women complete questionnaires about their sexual response and functioning before and after their participation in a group mindfulness program, most (if not all) aspects of sexuality improve significantly. The women's ratings of sexual desire for a partner may go from "almost never" to "almost always." Sexual satisfaction increases by 60 percent.

However, because the questions that make up these scales are often very brief, these questionnaires may not fully reflect participants' experiences or reveal important information about how mindfulness has affected them. Researchers may then turn to other means of discovering how participants were affected by the program and, specifically, whether those statistically significant improvements were also *clinically meaningful* to the women.

In each of our controlled scientific studies of mindfulness as it is applied to a variety of sex-related concerns, an independent investigator—someone not directly involved in leading the mindfulness sessions—asks participants to share anonymously what they liked and did not like about their mindfulness experience and how they were affected, if at all. We keep this feedback anonymous to minimize bias: if the women knew that their names would be linked to their responses and that their own mindfulness group facilitator would be reading their feedback, they might filter or alter their feedback by, for example, being less likely to state that they found the groups boring or a waste of time.

Over the past decade we have compiled the feedback provided by our group participants. Here are a few examples of what they have told us:

"I didn't think that paying attention to my breath was going to make any dent in my longstanding sexual difficulties, but I was completely wrong! I learned that paying attention to the basic sensations of my body was key to improving my sexuality."

"I was entirely skeptical at the beginning when my doctor encouraged me to attend the mindfulness groups. After all, isn't sexual arousal dependent on physical events in the body? I now realize that healthy sexual arousal depends more on the mind than the body."

"It was so simple and right under my nose. Who would have thought that the answer I was looking for for years was right there? I just needed to be made aware of it."

"I joined the mindfulness program with the sole aim of increasing my sexual desire, but what I got was so much more than that. I discovered that my sexual desire was always there, but I needed to pay attention to it, and I also found that I became better at managing stress and anxiety in my life. It was such a gift to participate in this program!"

These testimonials are not captured in many of the standard questionnaires given in sex research. Sadly, our society places a premium on frequency measures: frequency of sex, frequency of orgasms, frequency of satisfying sexual events. The U.S. Food and Drug Administration (FDA), which approved Addyi, was more interested in the frequency of monthly satisfying sexual events than in how women *felt* about those events. But the women participating in our mindfulness programs did not talk about notches on a bedpost or number of orgasms. Instead, they described the impacts of mindfulness on their sexuality in a different way—one based on feeling more in tune, noticing feelings in a more intense way, and experiencing a deeper type of sexual desire and pleasure.

In the early days of our work, we delivered mindfulness in a four-session group program. Women asked for more. They wanted longer sessions and more sessions. They did not mind our suggestions that they practice mindfulness daily between our group sessions. When we adopted their suggestions and expanded the program to eight weeks, with 2¼ hours per session and up to forty minutes of daily meditation (unlike the recommended ten to fifteen minutes of daily practice in our earlier program), their commitment to the daily practice was unwavering. Many of the group leaders' beliefs that "busy women will not do this" were debunked. The women signed up, they showed up, and they wanted more. No matter how busy they were, the women were eager to do the exercises. Currently we have waiting lists for women wanting to join the groups. Every week I receive emails, tweets, and phone calls from women and health-care providers around the world wondering how they can participate in similar mindfulness groups for sexual desire located in their own city.

If you are a beginner to mindfulness and want to use this book as a guide to explore your own sexual desire, I encourage you to consume all of your meals for the next three days with more awareness. In the same way that you slowly and purposefully noticed sensations of the raisin, see if you can bring those same qualities of attention to your meals. This exercise will then serve as a building block for a series of other mindfulness exercises designed to put you more in touch with yourself, your body, and, ultimately, your sexuality.

CHAPTER 4

BECOMING AWARE
OF YOUR BODY

The body benefits from movement. The mind benefits from stillness.

SAKYONG MIPHAM, *Running with the Mind of Meditation*

HAVING ATTENDED MINDFULLY to their meals over several days, the women who participate in our group sessions at the University of British Columbia are then guided through a variety of mindfulness exercises using a different focus of attention during each one. After the eating meditation, they are guided through a twenty-to-thirty-minute Body Scan, which invites them to move their focus to various areas of the body and to take note of the sensations they experience in each area. They are then given an audiorecording of a forty-minute Body Scan to use daily at home. They are encouraged to track the date and time of their at-home practices, as well as any observations about or reactions to them.

Carving out the time to do the at-home exercises is one of the biggest challenges the women experience. They are already juggling jobs and a variety of other obligations, tasks, and responsibilities. Many have children or elderly parents who are dependent on them. We openly discuss their anticipated struggle with doing the at-home practices and brainstorm with other women in the group about strategies they have used to find the time for these exercises. For many of the women, the benefits of the exercises provide enough motivation for them to continue. During the Body Scan they notice that they can pay attention to sensations in a region of their body that they typically ignore: "I didn't realize that my back produced so many sensations. When I stop to notice them, I'm surprised at how nice they feel."

It is also worth noting that we refer to mindfulness as a "practice," and in so doing, we really intend two meanings. First, we are referring to it simply as an activity—treating it as a regular practice or activity, such as brushing your teeth every day. Second, we are also referring to it as an exercise that leads to proficiency—in cultivating present-moment awareness, without judgment, and ultimately in making changes in the brain. All of this requires practice—regular, habitual, and deeply embodied practice.

Fitness programs designed to get individuals from "fluff to fit" often use the "ninety-day" slogan in their marketing, based on the facts that building muscle is a slow process and that gains build on one another. However, once the ninety-day intensive program has been completed, the key to maintaining fitness is some type of maintenance practice in which you follow a less intense version of the original ninety-day intensive program.

Mindfulness may be thought of as working the same way. In most eight-week mindfulness-based stress-reduction programs, participants are encouraged to practice mindfulness for up to forty-five minutes a day. Once the program is over, many scale back to a more manageable schedule of slightly shorter daily mindfulness practices, or to forty-five-minute meditations a few times a week instead of daily.

During the Body Scan the women are also guided through an awareness of sensations in their genitals: "Just notice whatever sensations are present in the vulva, in the vagina, and in the hair-covered mons area. Notice if any thoughts arise as you pay attention to those areas, and whether the thoughts have any emotional tone to them—do you notice yourself feeling sad, frustrated, anxious, or anything else?" Rather than ignoring emotions, even the unpleasant ones, the women are guided to tune in to them. They are repeatedly told that "tuning in trumps tuning out." They therefore experience observing their own thoughts and emotions—worry, sadness, guilt—without acting on them. They learn that they can experience these emotions, whatever they are, without judging themselves or their situation. For some women, this may be the first time that they have not rushed to avoid negative emotions, or perhaps even not felt helpless in the face of them. They realize that there is room in the field of their awareness for positive, neutral, and negative sensations and emotions, and they can observe all of them. This is a powerful experience and provides the push to continue the at-home practices and to reaffirm their commitment to attending the eight weekly group sessions.

If you wish, you can now try the Body Scan, which has been adapted from mindfulness-based stress reduction (MBSR) and mindfulness-based cognitive therapy (MBCT) for women with sexual concerns. If you have practiced the Body Scan in the past, it is likely that you will find this version slightly different in that we spend as much time noticing sensations in the genitals, breasts, and other sexually sensitive parts of the body as traditional Body Scans do paying attention to the toes, the back, and the earlobes. The key to the Body Scan is to observe the sensations in the body in as much detail as possible and with equal interest in pleasant, unpleasant, and neutral sensations. In this practice you are not bringing up certain scenes in your mind from the past or engaging in mental imagery; you are simply observing what is happening in the present.

In the Body Scan you become aware of whatever sensations are present in different parts of your body in each passing moment and bring an accepting attitude to whatever arises in your field of awareness, looking at it clearly and seeing it as it is. It is important to keep in mind that as you take note of certain parts of the body, you may wish to create a new sensation there, or move that part of the body, or flex or relax a muscle, and so on, particularly if the feeling there is discomfort or pain. It is a natural human tendency to want things to be different from how they are right now. For this practice, however, your goal is not to change your experience or to become more relaxed. You are simply going to observe whatever sensations are there, with an open and accepting attitude.

The Body Scan

Before you begin, ensure that the room is a comfortable temperature, but not so warm that it could put you to sleep. Next, find a comfortable position in your chair, lie down on a yoga mat, or sit on a firm pillow on the ground. For some women, lower back support may be helpful. You may feel you want to close the eyes, but remember that this practice is about "falling awake," not falling asleep, so if you sense a tendency to doze off, try to keep the eyes open and fixed on a particular spot ahead of you.

1. Begin by bringing a general awareness to your posture, with your back in an upright, dignified position and your spine, neck, and head in alignment if you are sitting. If you are lying down, extend the top of your head and the bottoms of your feet, gently, in opposite directions.

2. For a few minutes, just become aware of your breathing. Notice the rate, depth, location, sounds, pressure, temperature, and other characteristics of your breathing. You are not manipulating your breath or trying to breathe deeper or differently. Your goal is just to pay attention. Also, there are no "correct" sensations to notice as you pay attention to the breath, or to other parts of the body for that matter. Whatever arises in your attention is worthy of paying attention to. You're going to just keep following the breath with your "mind's eye" for a few minutes.

3. After about a minute or so, move your attention down the left side of your body, all the way down to the toes of your left foot. This area—the individual toes, the spaces between the toes, and the points of contact between the toes and your sock, shoe, or floor—will be your new focus of attention.

4. Try to notice as many individual sensations as you can. For example, do you notice sensations of contact, tingling, moisture, itching, or warmth or coolness? You may detect that there are no prominent sensations when you try to focus on an area. That is fine too, and you can notice what it feels like to not notice sensations. The specific sensations are not important. Bring attention to the toes as they are. If you find that no sensations are present in this region, then just experience what's there. Experience the big toe as it is, and the little toe, and perhaps the toes in between.

5. After a minute or so of noticing the toes, and other regions of the left foot, move your attention up to the ankle, then to the lower leg, the knee, and the upper areas of the left leg, paying attention to the various sensations in every region. Remember that your goal is to simply observe, not to create any different sensations. Often many of us may lose focus and notice other sounds or thoughts, possibly even thinking to ourselves, "This is boring" or "Is this working?"

6. Next, focus on the right foot and leg, the chest, the back, the arms, the neck, and the head.

7. When you are ready, move your attention to the right hip and the left hip and the entire area of your pelvis, following these instructions:

8. Notice any sensations in your pelvis and lower abdomen, your buttocks, and your genitals, including sensations of contact with your chair, yoga mat, or floor.

9. Become aware of the region of your genitals, including sensations of warmth or weight, either mild or intense, whatever is there in this moment. You are not trying to create sensations or arousal but simply to notice.

10. Pay attention to the distinct areas of the genitals—the labia, the clitoris, the perineum, and maybe even the vaginal opening. As with other regions, there may be no sensations apparent to you, and that is fine. Spend some time just observing as your eyes remain closed.

If you do notice sensations, are they pleasant, unpleasant, or neutral? There may also be thoughts that come up, and as best as you can, simply allow even judgmental or critical thoughts to be there without reacting to them or judging yourself for having them. Bring the same gentle acceptance to thought sensations as you are bringing to any physical sensations.

11. Having now paid attention to all the individual regions of the body, you can next spend a few moments expanding your field of awareness to include your entire body, from the top of your head to the bottoms of your feet. Try to pay careful attention to the many individual sensations that arise and pass away within this larger field of awareness, wherever they may be located in the body. You can allow your attention to move fluidly from sensation to sensation, wherever they arise in the body, momentarily focusing on each one as it rises and fades. Spend a minute or two observing in this way.

12. As your practice comes to a close, deliberately form an intention to introduce movements into your fingers and toes, and before you move them, watch closely how that intention to move gets translated into the movement of those body parts. Pause for a moment. Next, make an intention to open your eyes, and then slowly allow that command to reach your eye muscles to open them. Pause. You can make any other movements you would like. Thank yourself for taking this time to bring a nonjudgmental awareness to your body, and remember that this state of awareness is accessible to you by simply attending to sensations at any time of the day.

BRINGING MINDFULNESS TO OTHER ACTIVITIES

IN OUR MINDFULNESS groups, we spend half of each group session engaging in a mindfulness practice together, then discussing what we observed and how this practice might be relevant to sexual response and sexual concerns. In between each weekly session, the women are also given specific body-awareness exercises to do at home. The Body Scan is practiced daily for approximately forty minutes. If forty minutes is challenging, we encourage the women to practice for as long as they can and then attempt to add on a few minutes the next time they practice. We also encourage them to bring their mindfulness to other activities involving awareness of their bodies. They are encouraged to have a shower or bath mindfully.

Bathing Mindfully

1. Take a bath or a shower. As you do so, notice particular parts of your body, such as your hands, arms, breasts, stomach, legs, and feet. Focus your attention on your body and let your thoughts simply "be as they are" in the background. Use all of your senses as you do this to enhance the experience. For example, notice the texture of your skin, its color, and what sounds or smells might emerge as you bathe.

2. Once you have finished and have dried off, spend a few minutes noticing yourself in a mirror. What can you appreciate about your body? (Think about function—not just appearance.) Are there parts of your body that give you a sense of pleasure or pride? Are there any parts of your body that you do not appreciate? Your body is alive. What does it feel like? Are there aspects of your body that deserve more attention? As you do this, notice any emotions you may be feeling, both positive and negative. It will

be important to leave this exercise with the feeling that your experience of your body is a balance of things you do like or appreciate and perhaps things you do not or wish were different. Throughout the rest of the day, be aware of your body as you engage in your daily routine.

Women often have distorted or inaccurate views of their own genital anatomy. "The vagina" is used to refer to the entirety of women's vulva, vagina, and genital regions, and this lack of precision, mixed with a general societal discomfort around talking about women's genitals, means that many women are not aware of the intricacies of their own genital anatomy. The myth that the vagina is the gateway to sexual pleasure continues to pervade our society, and many women (and their partners) are not aware of the wonderful complexity of the clitoris. Only a small segment of the clitoral hood and shaft protrude from the body and are visible to us; most of the body of the clitoris lies below the surface of the skin, invisible to a woman and her partner, and waiting to be discovered.

After providing some educational information about female anatomy in the group sessions, we encourage the women to go home and use a hand-held mirror to mindfully touch and explore their own body. They are encouraged to explore with curiosity, not with the intent of eliciting sexual arousal. For many women in our groups, this is their first "hands-on" opportunity to learn about and experience their own body. As thoughts or emotions such as fear and guilt arise, the women are encouraged to invoke their mindfulness skills of compassion and nonjudgment to experience everything that arises and unfolds, moment by moment.

I have seen many women walk away from this exercise with tears in their eyes and with an immense sense of gratitude for feeling that they had permission to look at their own genitals. This particular exercise provides an opportunity in a group session to talk about body image and its gripping effects on women's sexuality and their sense of their sexual self. As a group, we discuss the participants' current level of body esteem. Many of the women state that they feel tremendous shame about their bodies—that they do not undress in front of their partner, that they wear unflattering clothes to mask their shape, or that they avoid looking in mirrors. Often they will share stories of how their low body esteem affects their sexual interactions. They may move a partner's hand away from a part of their body that has an extra skin fold, or they may shorten or bypass kissing and caressing entirely out of fear that a partner feels a particular part of their body.

Week by week as our eight-session program continues, the women become immersed in both in-session and at-home daily mindfulness exercises. Many of the women attending these groups begin to experience improvements in their day-to-day life and interactions, and they react with less stress to typically stressful scenarios. Some of them report improvements in their mood, anxiety levels, and overall well-being.

THE CIRCULAR SEXUAL RESPONSE CYCLE

WE ALSO INTRODUCE the women to Dr. Rosemary Basson's circular sexual response cycle and the concept of responsive desire (Figure 1). This model of sexual desire normalizes a woman's lack of sexual desire at the beginning of a sexual encounter. Basson argues that beginning from a state of being "sexually neutral" is not only nonpathological but is also probably quite normal for couples in long-term relationships. Basson's model then identifies the need to consider reasons for sex that prompt a woman to be open to sexual advances or to initiate sexual activity on her own. A combination of a conducive context (a bedroom environment free from distractions) and appropriate sexual stimuli (the types of sexual touches, sounds, smells, and other triggers that "work" to elicit arousal for that particular woman) then blend to make the woman respond with sexual arousal. If she attends to the sexual arousal and enjoys it, this can open the pathway to sexual desire and, eventually, sexual satisfaction. In other words, this model states that a woman experiences first arousal and then desire, not the other way around.

Figure 1. Rosemary Basson's Circular Sexual Response Cycle emphasizing responsive sexual desire

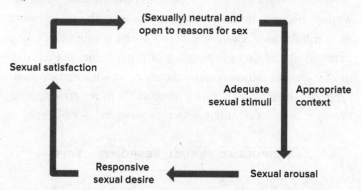

Countless inhibitors can break this cycle at any stage. For example, a woman who identifies no reasons for sex will have a hard time moving out of sexual neutrality. A distracting or negative environment, inadequate sexual stimuli, or touches, sounds, and smells that are off-putting for a woman can

interfere with the arousal-then-desire cycle. Basson has argued that mindfulness could be an ideal tool for mending the breaks in the cycle. For example, mindfulness skills may help a woman identify her reasons for engaging in sex or help her let go of negative thoughts or judgments about the environment. Mindfulness may also help her focus on the stimuli that could elicit sexual arousal. By paying attention in the present moment and nonjudgmentally, women may also take notice of the first signs of sexual arousal that they otherwise often miss because they are focused on the outcome.

Because Basson's model has helped countless women feel normal and not pathologized, we have integrated this model into our eight-session mindfulness program. Our own observation is that women can use the model to reinforce their reasons for practicing mindfulness. They can also identify where the breaks are in their own sexual response cycle and track which ones are mended as a result of cultivating their skills in mindfulness.

INTEGRATING TOOLS WITH
BUILDING SEXUAL AWARENESS

BY ABOUT WEEK Five, and after adopting mindfulness as a new regular practice (or even as a habit), the women in our groups begin to ask about how their acquired skills can be directly applied to their sex lives. It is at this point in the program that we introduce a "sexual sensations awareness meditation." We encourage the women to use a sexual aid of their choice as a way of first eliciting sexual arousal. There is a vast amount of literature on how erotica, vibrators, and sexual fantasy can elicit sexual arousal in women. In our mindfulness exercises we invite the women to consider them as tools to elicit arousal. For example, we offer the women guidance to create a fantasy in their mind for approximately five or ten minutes at home, stopping before they reach a high level of physical sexual arousal or climax. Immediately afterward, they listen to an audiorecording of a mindfulness exercise, where they are specifically guided to observe the sensations associated with arousal.

By combining the vibrator, erotica, or sexual fantasy with the sexual sensations awareness exercise, the women will be able to identify potential sexual feelings that they may otherwise ignore or not notice in their sexual encounters. And by not striving to have a particular response, to reach climax, or to have a certain type of sexual response that they think their partner expects them to have, the women experience freedom to feel whatever sensations arise—and this freedom from expectations leads them to tune in to a greater degree and ultimately boosts their sexual arousal. This exercise is an important step in unifying the mental and physical aspects of women's sexual excitement. First, though, here is a bit of background on sexual tools.

Sexual fantasy is a way of putting your mind in a sexual place, and it can help in those instances where your body is becoming sexually aroused but your mind is distracted and focused on nonsexual events or images. Most of us have used sexual fantasy at times. You may have caught yourself daydreaming while at work or while sitting on a bus. Unlike the dreams we have at night, our daydreams can be controlled—so you can create or re-create sexual scenes as you wish. Fantasy involves trusting yourself and letting your imagination go. Sexual fantasy is a normal, natural activity and a way of re-experiencing pleasurable or exciting situations, behaviors, and experiences. It is a way to express your creativity.

Some women admit to being hesitant to fantasize about someone other than their partner. Some worry that thinking about something is as bad as doing it. Guilt may arise during or after a fantasy, and for some women, guilt may prevent them from ever eliciting a fantasy. Many women use fantasy—it is a natural, healthy expression of your sexuality. Please consider fantasy as part of this exercise and give yourself permission to experiment a little bit. If you find you do not like fantasizing, you can always discontinue it.

Fantasies come in all shapes and sizes. Some fantasies that women have discussed include being with their partner but doing things they have never tried before or perhaps trying things in a new location, being with different lovers, or adopting a new identity. What makes fantasy exciting is that you can create a sexual scenario in your imagination that you might never act on in reality. The ability to imagine is the key to enjoying the sexual benefits of fantasy.

Vibrators can be a helpful way to augment your body's natural sexual response. What is your experience with vibrators? What are your attitudes toward using them? Some women are against their use because they think it is an artificial way to experience sexuality. If you feel this way, consider the vibrator as simply another option available to you, as a convenient and effective way to experience arousal, or as a way to make your sexual experience more interesting. Try to give yourself permission to consider this for the present moment. You do not need to make this a permanent part of your sexual repertoire in the future if you don't want to.

There are many different types of vibrators, in different shapes and sizes and with different settings and attachments. If you do not own one that you like already, do some shopping around to find the one that is right for you. You may wish to include your partner, if you have one, in your search. Many pharmacies and drugstores carry a variety of vibrators (often marketed as "personal massagers") in the contraceptive or family planning aisle.

The use of erotic materials such as movies, books, or works of art can help you connect with your sexual feelings in the same way that fantasy and vibrators can. Almost all women show an automatic physical reaction to erotica. This fact surprises some women, and learning to recognize their arousal to erotica can take time. Research consistently shows that women are typically unaware of their body's sexual responses or perceive them in a very muted way. Some women detect physical sensations but feel indifferent toward them. Many women with sexual difficulties may have negative feelings about being aroused or believe that their body is betraying them.

What are your beliefs about erotica? What experience have you had with erotic materials? What positive and negative thoughts come to mind as you think about or experiment with erotica? Erotica is not the same as pornography, which is exclusively focused on eliciting sexual arousal, tends to adopt a male point of view, and often focuses on close-ups of genital penetration. Erotica creates a scene in which the actors may engage in dialogue or flirting, and there is a build-up of anticipation before any sexual contact begins. The camera angles are softer, the music tends to be less bombastic, and there is more time focused on the woman's pleasure. Many women who are turned off or offended by pornography enjoy erotica.

Erotica produced by female directors tends to focus more on the woman than most pornographic movies do. Female-made, female-focused films, such as those produced by Erika Lust and the late Candida Royalle, are gentler and more appealing to women's tastes. Some women describe watching them as being like watching any movie, except that it contains explicit sexual scenes.

Sexual Sensations Awareness Exercise

For this exercise to create awareness of sexual sensations, I encourage you to explore different tools to find what pleases you.

If, like some of the women participating in our groups, you have concerns about using a sexual tool—fantasy, erotica, or a vibrator—in this exercise, it may help to remember that you are using it in a very specific manner. You are viewing or using it as a means of eliciting arousal and pairing it with a mindful exercise to observe how your body feels when you pay attention. If you don't feel ready to try this exercise, that is fine. You can continue to read this book and consider trying it in the future.

Once you have selected a sexual tool to use for this exercise, spend a few minutes engaging with it. As you do so, try to use all of your senses to fully immerse yourself in the experience. If you are using a fantasy, try to tune in to smells, touches, and sounds. If you are using a vibrator, try to really tune in to the qualities of the touch. You can shift the settings on the vibrator to elicit different types of vibrations and notice what each one feels like. If you are viewing erotica, try to fully observe the interaction between the actors, and if thoughts, beliefs, or judgments arise, try, just for the moment, to let those drift aside. After five to ten minutes of engaging with your fantasy, vibrator, or erotica, it is time to perform a body awareness exercise.

1. Lie on your bed in a balanced and relaxed position. Close your eyes, if that feels comfortable, and focus your attention on what is going on in your body. Observe your energy level, the sensations in your body as you are breathing, and perhaps sensations of the heart, such as the speed of your heart rate and the intensity of it. See if you can locate exactly where you feel your heart beating. Notice any sensations on your skin, perhaps tingling, warmth, or coolness.

2. Now focus your attention on your facial expression and sensations in your face. Then move the focus of your attention down the body, past your chest and breasts and belly, down to your pelvic area. You may wish to tune in to sensations in your genitals.

3. Allow your focus of attention to rest gently on the entire region of your vulva and vagina. Notice the individual sensations in this area of the body, as each emerges, lingers, and fades away. Try to become aware of how your genitals feel, moment to moment. There may be tingling, warmth, fullness, pulsation, or a lack of sensation. Observe each of these sensations without using your hands. Spend a few minutes observing in this way.

4. Try to move your attention even closer to the distinct sensations in different parts of the genitals. Can you detect sensations in the clitoris and the mons (hair-covered area) above the clitoris? Can you move your attention downward to sensations in your labia majora (outer lips)? What about the labia minora (inner lips)? What do you sense there? Do you notice sensations at the vaginal entrance and inside the vagina?

5. As you pay attention to these sensations, notice if you experience them as pleasant, unpleasant, or neutral. Do

you like the sensations and want to keep your attention focused on them, or do you dislike them and want to push those sensations away? Do these sensations "feel sexual" to you? Do you feel an urge to stimulate yourself further, maybe even to orgasm? Simply take note of what that urge feels like and continue to observe the sensations in your body without touching your body.

6. If you realize that you have forgotten about noticing sensations in your genitals because your attention was focused on the content of a thought or a story, simply note where your attention has gone and gently return it to the sensations in your genitals.

7. After paying attention to sensations throughout the genital region, you can now expand the focus of attention around the genitals to include a sense of your body as a whole as you continue to lie still with your eyes closed. You can allow your attention to rest on whatever sensation is most prominent, moment to moment, wherever it is located in your body. Continue to do this for a minute or two.

8. When you are ready, open your eyes.

WHO BENEFITS FROM MINDFULNESS FOR SEX?

HOW EFFECTIVE IS this mindfulness-based approach for improving women's low or altogether absent sexual desire? Does paying attention, deliberately and nonjudgmentally, make a lasting impact on women's sexual motivation? Since 2003, our large collaborative team has been evaluating the effects of mindfulness on women's sexuality in several hundred women. Mindfulness exercises were delivered in a variety of formats: individually or in groups; monthly, biweekly, and weekly; and face to face or online.

To capture how the women improve after participating in a mindfulness program, they complete questionnaires that ask about their desire for sex, their arousal, and their pleasure during sexual activity, as well as the frequency and intensity of their orgasms. They also fill out questionnaires about mood, anxiety, relationship satisfaction, and overall quality of life.

In addition, the women come into a private laboratory and self-insert a small sterile vaginal probe (the vaginal photoplethysmograph). While they watch two eight-minute excerpts from films—a neutral documentary on lei making in Hawaii and an erotic scene depicting kissing, caressing, foreplay, and sex—the probe measures their genital response. This provides an indirect measure of sexual arousal that does not reflect how a woman is feeling but shows how her body responds to erotic triggers.

The research reveals that these mindfulness-based groups significantly improve sexual desire, sexual arousal, orgasms, sexual satisfaction, and mood in women seeking treatment for low sexual desire. The women also experience markedly less distress about their low desire immediately after the program ends, and still feel that way when they are assessed half a year later. For some women, while their low desire has not changed with mindfulness treatment, they experience far less sex-related distress after it. The women who saw greater improvements in their ability to describe sensations and the women who had a more marked decline in negative mood were found to benefit the most from our group mindfulness sessions and to experience higher increases in sexual desire.

We also adapted the treatment for women survivors of childhood sexual abuse who, in addition to low sexual desire, experienced extreme phobic reactions to sex, even sex that was consensual in their current and otherwise happy relationships. Despite undergoing therapy for trauma symptoms and showing great improvement in post-traumatic stress disorder (PTSD) and other symptoms of anxiety, many of these women continue to struggle when it comes to sex. They enjoy kissing, touching, and mild caressing with their partners, but, once they start to become sexually aroused, some dissociate from the situation or experience flashbacks of being raped. This creates enormous distress for them, particularly in the context of being in an otherwise happy relationship.

We reasoned that if women could be encouraged to "ride out" their anxiety by staying in the present moment, and not catastrophizing that a (consensual) sexual encounter would end in disaster and disappointment, they might be able to tune in to their sexual arousal.

In a study we published in 2012, we noted that teaching sexual abuse survivors to mindfully pay attention to the present moment, to notice their genital sensations, and to observe "thoughts" simply as events of the mind led to marked reductions in their levels of distress during sex. In addition, the women had an increase in concordance (agreement) between their body's sexual arousal and their self-reported sexual arousal as they watched an erotic film. This seemed to be the clearest evidence we had collected that mindfulness works by integrating the body's and the mind's sexual responses.

Chapter 3 reviewed the research evaluating mindfulness in cancer survivors. The mindfulness program aimed at women with sexual dysfunction has also been applied to and extensively studied in survivors of gynecologic cancer who experienced sexual difficulties following their cancer treatment. Consider Mae's story.

Mae was diagnosed with stage II cervical cancer at the age of twenty-five. Given the stage of her cancer, she was advised to undergo a radical hysterectomy, in which the entire uterus, cervix, and the upper third of the vagina are removed. Like the majority of cervical cancer survivors who experience sexual difficulties after treatment, Mae had great difficulty becoming physically aroused. Whereas she had previously quickly become lubricated during kissing and petting with her boyfriend, after her radical hysterectomy she said she felt "dead down there," and in the two years since her cancer treatment she felt that she had lost all sexual desire and arousal. She used copious amounts of lubricant just to allow vaginal penetration, but still found penetration uncomfortable. The quality of the sensations in her vagina was vastly reduced, and she likened genital touch to "feeling like my boyfriend is touching my elbow, not touching one of the most sensitive parts of my body." With the drop in her arousal also came less motivation for sex, and she began to avoid potential sexual encounters by going to bed at different times from her partner or by faking a headache.

Mae learned the Body Scan meditation first and practiced bringing her awareness to the sensations in the different parts of her body in a way she had never done before. She then learned to systematically guide her attention from an array of thoughts to the sensations in her arms, hands, legs, feet, and toes. She described the sensations aloud to the other women in the group. Over time, and as she felt more comfortable tuning in to her body in a nonjudgmental way, she realized it was time to apply these skills to her sexual encounters with her boyfriend. During sex with her boyfriend, Mae was often bombarded with thoughts such as "I will never respond like I used to," "I'm no longer sexual," "My body is dead," and "My boyfriend will leave me unless I regain my sexual response." Understandably, these catastrophic thoughts gave rise to significant anxiety for her both leading up to and during her sexual encounters. She also worried that there was nothing she or her doctors could do to improve her functioning. The more she worried, the more depressed she felt, and she felt guilty that her partner was too young to be resigned to be in a sexless relationship.

In group sessions, and with the support of the other women in the group, Mae worked at relabeling these distressing thoughts as mental events—just thoughts the brain creates rather than statements about reality or predictions about the future. Adopting this dispassionate stance toward her thoughts helped Mae to fend off the sadness, guilt, and anxiety that accompanied sexual activity and allowed her to remain present. She started to focus mindfully on genital sensations during her partner's light touching, and observed that her belief that her "genitals were dead" was not accurate. With the expectation of sexual activity removed, over time Mae could touch and be touched on her vulva and vagina, and meditate fully on the emerging sensations. It was as if her vagina and vulva had awakened.

As Mae regained awareness of the feelings in her genitals, she realized that the surgery had not removed all of her ability to respond to touch, even though the surgical changes to the length of her vagina had led to discomfort with deep penetration. Although her response was not as intense as it had been before, Mae did find that by paying attention to the sensations and guiding her mind onto her body, she experienced a satisfaction in her arousal that she had taken for granted before her surgery. By learning about Basson's concept of responsive desire, Mae also no longer worried when she did not feel desire at the beginning of a sexual encounter. Instead, she focused on triggers for her sexual arousal, and then used mindfulness to pay attention to those sensations. In so doing, her desire for sex emerged *during* the encounter. As her pleasure from sexual touch increased, her sexual desire increased also, and she was now initiating sex for the first time in two years.

A number of studies have now evaluated mindfulness for addressing sexual concerns in cancer survivors. Compared with a control group of women who waited for three months before receiving mindfulness treatment, the women who completed the mindfulness meditation program earlier had significantly improved sexual desire, arousal, lubrication, orgasm, and sexual satisfaction. In one study, survivors who became sexually aroused while watching an erotic film in a controlled laboratory environment reported that they experienced more genital arousal than before their mindfulness training. When the program was adapted for online delivery, the women who participated experienced similar increases in sexual response and satisfaction to those of the women who participated in the face-to-face treatments. Furthermore, when the women were assessed six months later, the improvements in their sexual functioning remained, suggesting that the treatments have lasting effects.

What happened to Sarah after she completed the eight sessions of our mindfulness program? After learning mindfulness skills and adopting a regular daily practice, Sarah realized that she, like so many women, erroneously believed that sexual desire should be automatic and that sexual activity should come naturally and easily. Therefore, when the touch she received from Seojun did not elicit her "typical" level of response, she believed that she was broken sexually and that she and Seojun were not a good match. On top of that, Sarah realized that apart from the early days of her relationship, when she was fully in tune with Seojun and the sexual activities they were engaged in (particularly if they involved an element of excitement like kinky sex), she was often distracted during sexual activity.

As she took note of this and began to guide her mind fully back to the encounter, and to the unfolding physical sensations, she realized that she could enhance her sexual responsiveness by simply paying attention. Over and over she told herself, "Let the distractions be," without needing to extinguish them or force her attention far away from them. With time, Sarah learned to remain with her growing sexual feelings even in the midst of having other thoughts and emotions. She exercised compassion by telling herself, "Just this moment," and she learned to let go of her judgment of Seojun and of herself. With time, Sarah experienced sexual desire in a way that felt robust and lasting. She learned to cultivate a sense of wanting again. And her confidence in her relationship with Seojun also flourished.

By paying attention to what is already there, mindfulness may be the best way of re-establishing sexual desire and passion in relationships.

CHAPTER 5

"YOUR ATTENTION, PLEASE!"

The most precious gift we can offer anyone is our attention.
When mindfulness embraces those we love, they will bloom like flowers.

THICH NHAT HANH, *Living Buddha, Living Christ,* 2007

WHERE ARE YOU right now? Perhaps you responded with "sitting in my reading chair" or "lying in my bed." But what I mean is, where is your mind right now? As you read the words on this page, are you partially going over your to-do list, thinking about what to make for dinner, planning the weekend, or replaying the events of the day? If so, you are not alone. We are increasingly pulled in a multitude of directions, and there are many demands on our attention.

Think about the events of your day for a moment. How many times did you feel like your attention was drawn to attend to different tasks simultaneously (for example, eating dinner while reading the paper while having a conversation)? I experience this regularly when each of my three children asks me (different) questions at the same time. Now, how many times today did you fully attend to just one task? Could you stand in line at the grocery store and just take note of all of your sensations while waiting (and resist the urge to check your phone or open a magazine)?

Growing up, if I stubbed my toe on the leg of the coffee table while running in the house, my father would say to me, "Where were you?" And I would reply, "Dad, you saw where I was! I was running in the living room." To which he would reply, "But... *where* were you?" At the time I would get very frustrated, and for a while I thought my father had a hearing problem. But now I realize that what he was asking me was, "Lori, where was your attention as you were sprinting across the living room floor?"

"I AM AN EXPERT MULTITASKER"

OUR ATTENTION WANDERS like a puppy, drawn to whatever intrigues us at any given moment. Sometimes we find ourselves lost in thought for minutes (or even hours) when we were meant to be engaged in something else. How quickly our mind moves from one thought to the next, in a seeming sea of thoughts that take us out of the present moment. I'm intrigued when I hear someone make light of this. And I'm mystified when I hear someone boast about their "ability" to multitask. "I'm very good at having a conversation with someone at a party while at the same time scanning the crowd for people I know and listening to other conversations." But science shows us that there are costs associated with this type of multitasking.

Let's take text messaging and driving as an example. A meta-analysis (a type of analysis that combines the results of many studies that have investigated the same topic) of twenty-eight large controlled studies evaluating the effects of texting and driving found large and consistent effects across the studies. Whether you only type on your phone or type and read while driving, there is a substantial negative effect on eye movements, reaction time to road hazards, lack of control of vehicle position on the road (as drivers reach to grab phones or drive with a single hand), and number of crashes. Several experts have even noted that texting while driving is more dangerous than talking on a cellphone, driving drunk, or driving while under the influence of marijuana.

The meta-analysis concluded that the reason behind the fatal effects of texting was a driver's impaired ability to adequately direct attention to the road. In fact, the science of attention has shown that our attention cannot actually be in different places at the same time; we shift our attention between tasks. Each time our attention shifts, there is a cost, known as cognitive load. As the study on "infomania" discussed in Chapter 1 revealed, the "cost" of repeatedly shifting attention between different tasks in frequent succession is roughly the same as a 10-point drop in IQ.

Perhaps you know someone who proudly claims to be able to pay attention to two activities simultaneously and can fully recall the details of each activity afterward. They are actually shifting their attention rapidly from one activity to the next, and during each of these shifts, they momentarily lose some cognitive abilities, meaning they are more likely to make errors and take longer to complete their tasks.

ATTENTION AND SEXUAL FUNCTIONING

FOR MANY DECADES, sex researchers have believed that attention is a critical aspect of sexual functioning. In the 1950s and 1960s, Masters and Johnson tested how the body responds during sexual activity and increasing levels of sexual arousal. To do this, they had couples engage in sexual activity in their laboratory with sensors to measure physiological response attached to various parts of the participants' bodies. They noticed that those who engaged in spectatoring and criticized themselves for their sexual performance were less connected to their body's response, and their emotional reactions consisted of fear and anxiety. Because sensate focus involves paying attention to touch and continually redirecting the focus of attention away from worrisome thoughts and back to the body's sensations, Masters and Johnson believed that it was this redirecting of attention that made sensate focus so successful. Studies evaluating their approach found that 95 percent of couples improved and that they were still benefitting when they were evaluated up to five years later. Masters and Johnson's work led scientists to believe that attention was a key factor in sexual arousal and that inattention was a potent inhibitor of a healthy sexual response.

Since Masters and Johnson's seminal work, other researchers have conceptualized additional models of sexual response in hopes of providing a framework for understanding how it unfolds and for identifying what factors might get in the way of sexual arousal. One of the more popular models of sexual response, which is called the incentive motivation model and which also emphasizes the role of attention, argues that like emotions, sexual response is evoked in response to a certain trigger. When we are deprived of food or drink, internal mechanisms in our body motivate us to eat or drink in order to maintain homeostasis—and to survive. But desire for sex does not operate on a deprivation model. For years, though, experts believed that it did—they believed that the longer one went without sex, the more internal pressure would build until it was "released" through sexual activity and homeostasis was restored. Although some believe that the longer we go without sex the more we want it, the experience of many women with low sexual desire is the opposite—the longer they go without sex, the more they become convinced that they could live without it, and their motivations for sex become more focused on appeasing an unhappy partner than on satisfying their own sex drive.

There is much more evidence now that sexual response is like other emotional responses, that it is elicited *in response* to some type of trigger. We feel happy when we have a pleasant thought or when someone does something that makes us feel good. Happiness does not "reside" within our mind (or body); rather, it occurs in response to something in the environment. In the same way, sexual response is elicited by a trigger. Perhaps the trigger is a thought, or a visual cue, or something that another person says or does. The range of cues that can elicit sexual response varies greatly across individuals, and how effectively these cues elicit a sexual response may change over one's lifetime or the duration of a relationship. Remember that quirky thing a partner did that used to drive you wild (in a good way) when you started dating? And then, several years into the relationship, drove you crazy (in a not so good way)? This is an example of how triggers, and our response to them, can change over time.

The incentive motivation model also states that your sexual reaction is influenced by, among other things, your biology, hormones, and neurotransmitters, which are chemical messengers released by the brain. Attention is critical for what you *do* in response to the sexual trigger: attentional mechanisms, which are largely tied to memory, determine whether you attach a sexual versus a nonsexual meaning to the trigger based on your past experiences with that type of trigger. Attention is also necessary for generating a response to the trigger—both a genital response and a mental response ("Am I feeling excited/aroused/turned on? Or neutral/unexcited/turned off?"). It is the combination of your biological predisposition, which includes the activities of hormones and neurotransmitters, and an effective trigger that has a sexual meaning attached to it that then elicits a sexual response. Attention allows you to tune in to those sexual triggers and elicits your memory of how similar cues evoked a sexual response in the past. Attention to the signs of physical sexual arousal is then transmitted to the brain, which further processes information about the sexual cue, which, in turn, elicits more physical sexual response. In this way, attention is very important both for the initial response to a sexual trigger and for ongoing sexual arousal.

Over the last several decades, researchers have tested different aspects of the incentive motivation model, leading to a fundamental shift in how we understand sexual response in women (and in men). Notions of sexual response occurring "spontaneously" or out of the blue are simply outdated and do not follow from this evidence-based incentive motivation model. A collection of experimental studies by researchers around the globe have tested elements of this model, and clinicians have also become interested in how attention can be modified in order to facilitate incentive motivation and improve sexual response.

Since we know that attention is a key component of eliciting a sexual response, it follows that lack of attention is relevant to sexual problems. Is there evidence for this? Yes. In a 1976 study of sexually healthy male undergraduate students, researchers presented erotic stories through a headphone in one ear to the participants. Usually, such stories would pro-voke a robust erection and trigger mental feelings of being turned on. At the same time, increasingly complex math tasks were relayed to the other ear. The men's physical sexual arousal response was simultaneously measured with a penile strain gauge. The researchers found that as the mental math task increased in difficulty, the men's attention was diverted from the sexual stories, and the men had more and more difficulty getting an erection. In other words, the nonsexual instructions interfered with the potent sexual sounds and stories and nega-tively affected the men's sexual response.

Similar experiments have been carried out with women, and we have seen the same negative effects of distraction and inattention on sexual arousal. For example, in one study, half of the participants were shown an erotic film and then asked to add successive pairs of single-digit numbers shown on a screen and say the resulting total out loud. The other half of the participants watched the erotic film alone. The women who were given the math task reported significantly reduced sexual arousal and were also shown to have significantly reduced physiological sexual arousal.

During sex, have you ever moved your partner's hands away from your "trouble spots" or asked to have sex with the lights out? Many women report having negative thoughts about their bodies or their sexuality during sex ("What if I don't respond? Will my partner be upset if I don't have an orgasm?"), and these can pull attention away from the sexual cues and impede sexual functioning. Although women in gen-eral report many types of these negative thoughts, the more common ones relate to concerns about body image, lack of erotic thoughts, and thoughts about sexual abuse that some of them had endured.

Research suggests that a woman's negative thoughts about her body pull her attention away from erotic triggers (such as focusing on pleasurable touch or looking at an engaged and turned-on partner) and contribute to a lack of sexual arousal and desire. Perhaps you have had similar negative thoughts during sex. If so, can you recall what effect it had on your sexual arousal, your motivation, and your level of satisfaction during and after the encounter? Have you ever experienced what felt like an abrupt shutting down of your sexual response during an encounter? What did you do as a result? Research shows that women with distressing low sexual desire are significantly more likely to consider themselves failures and to disengage ("When will this be over?") than women without sexual concerns. Therefore, a momentary lapse in attention and a resulting lack of sexual response can trigger a cycle of catastrophic thoughts and worries that lead to further attention being pulled away from sexual cues.

Scientists have measured the effects of attention on sexual response in a university laboratory setting. In the dot detection task, for example, two images are presented on a computer screen for a fraction of a second, and then a small white dot appears where one of the images had been. Participants saw either two neutral images (showing objects such as kitchen utensils) or a neutral image paired with an erotic image (showing intercourse or oral sex, for example). They were then told to press a red key if the dot was presented on the left side of the screen and a blue key if the dot was presented on the right. The dot was presented randomly on either side of the screen. The time taken to detect the dot when it was shown where the sexual image had been was recorded against the time taken to detect the dot when it was where the neutral image had been.

Participants who showed higher levels of sexual desire on a questionnaire before the experimental task began were slower to detect the dot in the sexual location than the one in the neutral location, whereas those reporting lower levels of sexual desire on the questionnaire were slower to detect the dot in the neutral location. The researchers reasoned that the sexual images were less novel for the participants with higher levels of sexual desire, so they were able to move their attention more quickly from the sexual location to the starting position than those in the low-sexual-desire group, who may have found the sexual material more novel. This study provided evidence that attention influences women's sexual desire. In another test of attention, this one involving women with a clinically diagnosed sexual desire disorder, the researchers found that in contrast to women who did not have low desire, those with low desire did not associate the sexual images with positive feelings. In other words, it was not necessarily that the women with low desire paid less attention to the sexual triggers but that when they did pay attention, fewer positive emotions were elicited.

Not only does lack of attention impede sexual functioning, but where a woman focuses her attention during sex can also affect her sexual response. Research has found that when male partners focus on their partner's response, especially if the partner has a strong sexual arousal response, the man's physical arousal is increased—he has a stronger erection. In other words, paying attention to a partner's increasing excitement may heighten one's own attention to those sexual signs and further strengthen one's sexual arousal. Research has also shown, however, that if the man's focus is on himself, his physical response is lower. In other words, if he worries about his own response and doesn't notice his partner's increasing excitement, his erection trails off.

But there is a particular nuance to this effect of self-focus on sexual arousal. Dutch researchers examined this experimentally by focusing a camera on participants while they watched a sexually explicit film and measuring their sexual response. The researchers found that the camera interfered with sexual arousal among those participants who were high in self-consciousness but led to improved sexual response among those participants who were low in self-consciousness. The researchers speculated that high levels of self-focus may lead one to monitor their responses in a negative manner and that low levels of self-focus might prevent adequate attention being paid to sexual cues—in both cases dampening response. A moderate level of self-focus, one in which a person is aware of their body and internal sensations, but not hypervigilant to them, may be essential for sexual response.

The women I see in my clinical practice who have a high degree of self-focus often describe negative and judgmental thoughts, and this likely explains why their high self-focus is actually counterproductive to their sexual response. However, if their self-focus can be altered so that it is not self-critical, it could facilitate their sexual response. Thus, it seems that the *type* of self-focus matters. It also means that altering the nature of the self-focus may be therapeutically helpful. It truly is about being aware and noticing subtle changes in sensation, but letting go of the negative interpretations of what one is sensing.

MANIPULATING ATTENTION

CAN ATTENTION BE manipulated experimentally in order to boost sexual response? Yes. In 2009, Australian researchers at Deakin University asked one group of women viewing a sexually explicit video to imagine themselves as the woman in the video along with a partner of their choice. Another group of participants was asked to watch the explicit scene as observers who also critically evaluated the sexual interactions. Women who watched the film as if they were a participant, and therefore focused more attention on the film, reported a significantly higher degree of sexual arousal and more positive feelings about the film than those who watched it as observers and therefore focused less attention on it.

Attention can also be manipulated by giving participants different instructions or feedback about how they are responding sexually. In a study that used an auditory pitch as a measure of the woman's level of sexual arousal, women were instructed to either increase or decrease the pitch by altering their level of sexual arousal. In other words, they could consciously increase the volume of the pitch by increasing their level of genital sexual response. Women were able to reduce their physical sexual arousal (and decrease the pitch) quite easily, and with more ease than they were able to increase the pitch (and therefore increase their physical sexual arousal). This finding provides support for the speculation that women can control their physical sexual arousal response.

Another factor that can increase attention, and thus sexual arousal, is novelty. Showing women the same sexually explicit film over and over leads to a decline in their genital arousal, while introducing a novel erotic stimulus, which increases their attention, restores their genital response to a higher level.

In a Canadian study in 2015, researchers asked participants how much attention they paid to a variety of ninety-second sexually explicit films. Although men attracted to men and women attracted to women reported paying more attention to films depicting same-sex encounters than films depicting opposite-sex encounters, heterosexual women reported paying the same amount of attention to the opposite-sex and same-sex erotica. Overall, there was a moderate degree of association between their level of attention to the films and their level of sexual arousal—providing further evidence that attention is important for sexual response.

CAN MINDFULNESS IMPROVE ATTENTION?

WE THEREFORE HAVE abundant evidence that distraction and inattention can interfere with sexual arousal and that people with sexual difficulties may have attention impairments that contribute to their sexual concerns. The incentive motivation model provides evidence that attention is a key factor in evaluating a sexual trigger and determining whether one will experience sexual arousal or not. But is there evidence that improving attention can improve sexual functioning in women with problems related to sexual desire or arousal? The answer to this is partially yes. And can mindfulness be one effective means of increasing attention and therefore boosting sexual function? The answer to this is most definitely yes.

When we look at other patient populations that have received mindfulness training, there is indeed evidence that mindfulness improves attention. As these patients practice mindfulness, they are continually reminded to catch their attention when it drifts off and to gently and compassionately guide it back to a particular target, whether that focus is the breath, the body, or a raisin in their mouth: "Focus your attention on your breath. Notice when your attention has been drawn elsewhere and gently guide your attention back to the sensations associated with breathing." The instructions in mindfulness are gentle and meant to inspire a spirit of self-compassion rather than judgment. (For example, instead of thinking, "What is wrong with me that my attention is all over the place?" thinking, "Oh look, there goes my curious attention again; come back here.")

There is scientific evidence that participants following mindfulness training perform better on laboratory measures of attention. One such measure is the Stroop test, a neuropsychological test in which words are presented in different colors and participants are instructed to say the color that the word is printed in rather than the word itself. What makes this test difficult is that the word is a color that is different from the color it is shown in. For example, the word "green" might be printed in pink, so one must say "pink" and not "green." The Stroop test is a common measure of attention used in research as well as in clinical practice to identify problems in the frontal lobes of the brain. In order to perform the Stroop test accurately, brain areas involved in color perception must be activated while brain areas involved in reading must be deactivated. Attention is one of the skills required to perform the Stroop test accurately and quickly.

Following mindfulness training, participants perform the Stroop test more quickly and accurately (that is, they do not read the word but say the color it is printed in) than they did before the training. And areas of the brain centrally involved in executive attention—namely, the anterior cingulate cortex—are significantly more active in experienced meditators than nonmeditators.

A 2007 study from the University of Pennsylvania compared three groups of participants to ascertain whether previous experience with mindfulness affected attention or not. The first group had no experience in meditation before participating in an eight-week mindfulness-based stress reduction (MBSR) program. Members of this group were taught to choose a focus of attention (such as the breath) and concentrate on it for the full duration of the practice. When their mind wandered (which happens often), they were instructed to notice the mind wandering and redirect their attention back to their breath.

In the second group, experienced meditators attended a thirty-day meditation retreat during which they practiced meditation for up to twelve hours a day. Unlike the mindfulness-based stress reduction group, which focused on a specific point of attention, retreat attendees focused on whatever came to their attention, whether it was a bodily sensation, the breath, sounds, or thoughts.

The third group consisted of participants who had never meditated before and who received no mindfulness training during the study.

The three groups were then measured on three different aspects of attention. The first, known as alert attention, refers to maintaining a vigilant state of readiness. The second, known as orienting attention, directs attention to a particular location. The third aspect of attention, known as conflict monitoring, helps to prioritize competing tasks. All participants then took part in a study of reaction time in response to images on a computer screen, and some of the images included a distracting picture on the screen. The researchers found that the experienced meditators made fewer mistakes in detecting the visual target on the screen, despite the presence of distractions, and were faster than those who had never meditated. Also, after the eight weeks of mindfulness training, the participants had improved their ability to focus on the target image (showed better orienting attention) and to keep their attention there. The long-term meditators also showed evidence of better receptive attention than the less experienced and inexperienced meditators.

How did this happen? The researchers explained that the practice of repeatedly engaging attention, moving attention, and disengaging it leads to shifts in the parts of the brain involved in attention. In other words, mindfulness changes the brain to promote improvements in attention.

THE BRAIN: OUR MOST POWERFUL SEX ORGAN

UNDERSTANDING HOW MINDFULNESS affects sexual desire in women means that we need to look a little closer at how mindfulness affects the brain. After all, the brain truly is the most powerful sex organ, and a powerful physical sexual response cannot compensate for a disengaged brain when it comes to enjoying sex.

We have considered some of the different mechanisms that may explain why mindfulness improves sexual desire, and I would argue that if mindfulness is to have a longstanding effect on sexual functioning for women, there needs to be evidence that it affects the brain in those areas that are directly involved in sexual desire. Although only a few studies of brain imaging have been carried out in women with low sexual desire, there is evidence for differences in brain activity between those who complain of low sexual desire and those who do not. For instance, in a study looking at functional magnetic resonance imaging (fMRI) in women with clinically significant low sexual desire, the women with low desire were found to have less brain activation in the occipital cortex and the middle occipital gyrus than those in a control group. They also had more activation in the left inferior parietal lobe, the medial frontal gyrus, and the basal ganglia. (See Figure 2.)

Figure 2. Cross-section of the brain showing the basal ganglia and image of the major lobes of the brain

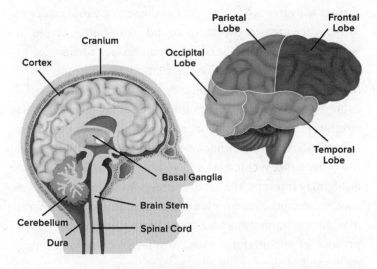

This means that the parts of the brain that were more active in women with low desire are associated with attending to, reflecting on, and making inferences about one's own emotional and mental states and those of others. This finding may help explain why women with low desire spend more time monitoring and evaluating their own sexual responses than attending to sexual cues.

This research has also shown that women with low desire have more activation in the lateral orbitofrontal cortex—which is associated with judgments about feelings—while watching erotic films. This area of the brain also controls our ability to suppress emotional responses. If a woman was having a negative reaction to a clip from an erotic film, this area of the brain would normally inhibit that emotional reaction. But this inhibitory function does not take place in a woman with low desire, allowing her to feel the full intensity of her negative emotions. For a woman with more robust sexual desire, it is possible that her feelings of sexual arousal may offset any negative emotions that are activated while she watches the sexually explicit scene.

Another area of the brain found to be more active in women with low desire is the putamen, an area that processes facial expressions. It is possible that when watching erotic films, women with low desire may interpret the actors' facial expressions negatively. For example, they may be more likely to interpret a quizzical look as registering disgust or aversion rather than reflecting either a neutral or positive emotion. On the other hand, women who have no concerns about sexual desire may interpret the facial expressions as conveying pleasure or other positive emotions. It is possible that mindfulness may directly target this area of the brain through the regular practice of encouraging women to let go of negative judgments and to observe the intricacies of sensations.

Whether it is for the treatment of chronic pain, stress, or arousal, mindfulness can be used to tune in instead of tuning out and to bring our full awareness to these bare sensations— moment by moment. And when we do so, we live better, fuller, more sexually fulfilling lives.

DESIRE AND DEALING WITH DISTRACTIONS

THE BRAIN IS responsible for attending to a sexual trigger, for associating it with positive sexual memories, for triggering the motivation for a sexual encounter, for eliciting a sexual response, and for ensuring that the body continues to respond to a sexual stimulus. It follows, therefore, that attention training through mindfulness may be part of the recipe for cooking up sexual desire. Let's see how this applies to Barbara.

Barbara is a thirty-two-year-old single lesbian woman who sought treatment for her lack of desire and sexual excitement. Barbara has had several sexual relationships, and her motivation for sex consistently dwindled when her relationships approached the six-month mark. Before that point, Barbara would enjoy the novelty of a new sexual partner and learning about each other's preferences. She was exploratory in the bedroom and was not shy to ask a partner to stimulate her in a particular way. As the months progressed, however, Barbara would find herself putting less effort into sex, and her attention would move toward sounds in the room, such as a ticking clock, and thoughts about the next day, and she would become disengaged sexually. "Sometimes while we have sex," she says, "I don't even notice when my partner has reached an orgasm."

Barbara took her dwindling motivation for sex as a sign that the relationship was doomed and would end the relationship at that point. But she also noticed a similar lack of attention in other areas of her life. During conversations, if the content was not interesting to her, she would drift into thinking about other things. Sometimes she would have almost no recollection of what she and a friend had talked about. "As long as things are novel," she said, "I'm interested, but I get bored easily, so the activities I do, the conversations I have, the things I see, must be changing, or my attention wanders." Barbara also wondered if she might have an underlying attention deficit problem, as her difficulties sustaining attention affected many aspects of her life.

Does Barbara's low level of motivation for sex mean that she has a sexual dysfunction? Probably not. However, her inattention to sexual stimuli means that her brain's processing of those stimuli is interrupted. She may be looking at something sexual, or even engaging in a sexual act, but because her mind is not paying attention to the sexual aspects of those events, those sexual cues are not registered in her brain as being sexual. Barbara's physical response becomes similarly blocked, the outcome is not rewarding, and her subsequent motivation for sex is understandably negatively affected.

Through training in mindfulness, Barbara learned to observe distracting thoughts as passing events of the mind. In the early stages of her practice, she noticed that her mind wandered off at least a hundred times during a ten-minute meditation practice. Although sometimes she would catch herself only after several minutes of being immersed in her thoughts, over time she learned to notice her mind wandering much more quickly and would redirect her attention back to her meditation practice. Barbara found it useful to label her thoughts as a "wandering mind" instead of paying attention to the specific thoughts, and this helped her redirect her attention before getting wrapped up in the contents of her thoughts. Barbara practiced this for a month, using her breath and her body as the focus of her attention. Then she began to experiment with this approach during sexual interactions.

Barbara noticed that "wandering mind" tended to set in as the novelty of her sexual experiences faded—around the six-month point in a relationship. In the past, she would automatically engage in catastrophic thinking that this meant there was lack of chemistry between her and her partner. Using mindfulness, she began labeling these worries "imagined catastrophes" as soon as she noticed them. In doing so, she was able to create some space between herself and these thoughts and to recognize that they were just mental events. She learned that she did not have to get automatically swept away by those thoughts.

In her mindfulness practice, and eventually in her sex life, Barbara no longer became absorbed into her stream of thoughts and was able to redirect her attention back to the physical sensations she was experiencing in the moment. With practice, she learned that even familiar touches and sexual behavior could continue to be exciting when she paid attention. She observed that arousal is not a static "on or off" phenomenon but rather a multitude of different sensations that are continually changing. As she paid closer attention to the sensations, her attention to them increased, as did her pleasure and enjoyment of sex. Barbara realized that her experience of arousal and pleasure was far more dependent on her level of attention than on any notions of pre-existing chemistry between her and a partner.

Barbara was thrilled that learning to cultivate attention was under her control, and she took great pleasure in feeling sensations in sex that she had not felt before. She also used mindfulness in her work environment—for example, during meetings, where she had the habit of drifting off and missing important conversations—and she began to feel more engaged in her social interactions. Finally, she mindfully addressed her belief that attention deficit/hyperactivity disorder made it impossible for her to pay attention and came to see even this as a passing event of the mind.

"Thoughts that arise are about as important as what you ate for dinner three nights ago." This is a statement that Jon Kabat-Zinn often makes to participants in his mindfulness groups as they struggle to carry out their mindful practices despite being distracted by random, and perhaps not so random, thoughts, such as "Why am I here? Will this really help to give me my sexual desire back? How on earth is paying attention to my breath relevant to my sex life?" When such thoughts arise among the women participating in our groups, we gently guide them to bring a kind curiosity to their thoughts by first noticing what kind of thought it is—for example, a planning thought, a memory, a judgment—and then to return to the practice they were doing before the thought captured their attention.

In our mindfulness practice, we try to observe thoughts rather than engage with their content. And unlike cognitive behavioral therapy (CBT), another effective psychological treatment described earlier in this book, a mindful approach to thoughts does not involve challenging or changing thoughts. And it certainly does not entail ignoring that the thoughts are there. You need to be aware of when you are engaging in the content of your thoughts and be able to switch your way of paying attention to them so that they can be observed rather than engaged with. Scientists refer to this process as "metacognition," or watching yourself thinking.

In mindfulness practice we do not suppress thoughts or attempt to modify them in any way. Many people misunderstand the instructions and make the mistake of thinking that meditation requires them to shut off their thinking or their feelings. They somehow hear the instructions as meaning that if they are thinking, it is "bad," and that a "good meditation" is one in which there is little or no thinking. Thinking is not bad; nor is it even undesirable during mindfulness practice. What matters is whether you are aware of your thoughts and feelings during meditation and how you handle them. Trying to suppress them may result in more tension and frustration. Mindfulness does not involve pushing thoughts away or walling yourself off from them to quiet your mind. You simply make room for them, observe them as "thoughts," and let them be, with an attitude of curiosity and acceptance.

Kabat-Zinn and other mindfulness leaders encourage us to consider thoughts as the by-product of the brain, a bodily organ just like the skin cells produced by the skin, bile produced by the gallbladder, or carbon dioxide produced by the lungs. If you can view thoughts simply as the by-product of your brain's daily activity, they begin to lose their dominance and importance, and then they can be experienced as having the same level of significance as any other sensations, such as the physical sensations of your belly while you breathe. Problematic thoughts ("I must not love my partner if I have no sexual desire") may still occur, but they can start to be viewed as just mental events, and their powerful influence is diminished.

To see how this works, you can try this mindfulness of thoughts meditation, which is adapted from our work with women with low sexual desire. You may choose to begin with five to ten minutes of mindfulness in which you focus on your body and/or your breath as described in earlier chapters. When you feel ready, you can move to focusing on thoughts using the following instructions as a guide.

Mindfulness of Thoughts

1. When you are ready, focus your attention so that the object of your awareness is your thoughts. Just as you focused awareness on different parts of your body, noticing whatever sensations arose, developed, and passed

away, so now, as best you can, bring your awareness to thoughts that arise in the mind in just the same way— noticing them as they arise, pass through the space of the mind, and eventually disappear. There is no need to try to make thoughts come or go. Just let them arise naturally, as you did with body sensations or breathing sensations as they arose and passed away.

2. Some people find it helpful to bring awareness to thoughts in the mind in the same way that they might if the thoughts were projected on the screen at the movie theater. You sit, watching the screen, waiting for a thought or image to arise. When it does, you pay attention to it as long as it is there on the screen, and then you let it go as it passes away. Alternatively, you might find it helpful to see thoughts as leaves being carried down a stream while you are sitting on the bank watching from a distance.

3. If any thoughts bring with them intense feelings or emotions, pleasant or unpleasant, you can notice the intensity of those feelings without a need to change them. Just simply notice how strong those emotions are.

4. If at any time you feel that your attention has become unfocused and scattered, or if it keeps getting drawn into your thinking or imaginings, you may want to notice where this is affecting your body. Often, when we don't like what is happening, we feel tension or tightness in the face, shoulders, or jaw. When this happens, you may want to "push away" your thoughts and feelings. Notice if any of this going on for you when some intense feelings arise. Then come back to the sensation of breathing and use this focus to anchor and stabilize your awareness.

5. Continue to observe your thoughts in this way for ten to twenty minutes.

6. At a certain point, let go of any particular object of attention, like your thoughts, your breath, or sounds in the background, and be open to whatever arises in the landscape of your mind and your body. Simply rest in awareness itself, effortlessly knowing whatever arises from one moment to the next. As you do this, you may become aware of sensations of breathing, sensations in the body, sounds inside and outside the room, thoughts, or feelings.

7. As best as you can, just sit, completely awake, not holding on to anything, not looking for anything, having no agenda whatsoever other than being fully awake and fully aware of your body here, resting in stillness.

8. And whenever you're ready, allow your eyes to open if they have been closed.

How did that practice go? Could you observe yourself thinking? If you did get swept away by the content of your thoughts, at what point did you notice this? Were you then able to haul yourself out of the stream and return to the bank, where you could once again watch your thoughts? Could you relate to the notion that thoughts are just transitory mental events that come and go? Next, consider the following: How might this way of paying attention to thoughts be relevant to your experience of sexual desire or difficulties with it?

Many of the women participating in our mindfulness groups recognize, after doing this mindfulness of thoughts practice, that they may be living in a seemingly never-ending stream of thoughts, coming out of the blue, one after another in rapid succession. Many people are greatly relieved to discover that they are not the only ones who find that their thoughts cascade through their mind like a waterfall, seemingly beyond their control.

But it is critical to remember that you are not your thoughts. Rather, you can relate to them just as you observe and notice other sensations in your body. Importantly, when you experience thoughts in this way, you learn that thoughts change from moment to moment, that some are pleasant while others are unpleasant, and that you are not defined by them. This discovery is quite a revelation for many people. It means that you can consciously choose whether or not to relate to your thoughts in a variety of ways that were not available to you before. One of the major barriers to women's use of mindfulness skills is their belief that they have no control over their wandering mind. In mindfulness practice, when you observe the multiple thoughts going through your mind as mental events, without getting engaged in their content, you stay firmly anchored in the present.

See if you can practice this mindfulness of thoughts exercise a few times throughout your day. Most people find it a challenging practice, so don't be hard on yourself if you get caught up in the content of your thoughts rather than watching them "from a distance." As with all of the exercises in this book, "practice" means that you must continually work at developing this skill. You may also consider trying this during sexual activity, a time when many women, and particularly those who experience sexual difficulties, are bombarded with thoughts, just as Barbara was. Try to notice judgmental thoughts that arise during sex as mental events, perhaps even telling yourself, "My mind seems especially active right now." Then gently guide your attention back to your body and back to the full constellation of sensations that bubble to the surface when your body and mind awaken sexually.

CHAPTER 6

HOW MINDFULNESS WORKS

Rather than viewing nonalignment of women's minds and bodies when it comes to sexual arousal as a sign that women may be consciously evading disclosure of sexual arousal, we should be focusing on understanding why the mind and body are not aligned.

MEREDITH CHIVERS, personal communication

IN CHAPTERS 3 and 4, we looked at how mindfulness skills improved Sarah's and Mae's sexual desire, arousal, and overall sexual satisfaction. In Chapter 5, we read about Barbara's struggles with inattention, which played a key role in her loss of sexual desire, and how mindfulness training improved her attention to sexual (and other) triggers. We have also considered some of the scientific evidence that mindfulness can significantly improve various aspects of sexual functioning, mood, and quality of life, and we know that modifying attention appears to be a key ingredient in that process. But one of the questions that scientists have not been able to definitively answer is "How exactly does mindfulness work to improve sexual functioning?" Could it be that people feel happier when they are mindful and that feeling happy contributes to greater sexual desire? Or perhaps mindfulness reduces stress and anxiety, leading to greater motivation to have sex.

As described in Chapter 5, at least some of the mechanisms underlying the benefits of mindfulness involve its effects on paying attention to the here-and-now, making practitioners of mindfulness more likely to tune in to sexual signals in their environment (and themselves) and therefore triggering feelings of being "turned on." Most of that discussion focused on paying attention to cues in the external environment; however, we can also improve our attention to cues from within our own bodies. And mindfulness training probably targets communication between the mind and the body, which is critical for sexual response. True, the body responds in a somewhat automatic manner in response to sexually explicit triggers, but this response is not likely to be enough to elicit motivation for sex. In other words, becoming turned on while watching a sexual scene in a film may not necessarily put you in the mood to have sex or prompt you to find a partner and start having sex.

CONCORDANCE: WHEN MIND AND BODY ARE IN AGREEMENT

PERHAPS YOU HAVE watched a sexually explicit scene in a movie or read an erotic passage in a book and noticed a physical arousal response (such as vaginal lubrication) despite having a neutral or even negative mental reaction. Perhaps you thought to yourself, "I don't find this scene sexy" or "I'm turned off right now," and yet your body was reacting in a manner that suggested it was sexually aroused. This is an example of sexual discordance, or disagreement between mental sexual arousal and physical sexual response. Discordance can happen in the other direction, too—that is, you may feel sexually turned on mentally but have little or no accompanying physical sexual response; the mind is ready for action, but the body says "No!" Many women experience discordance after some types of pelvic surgery that alter the sensitivity of the genitals to touch, leaving them with a lack of sensation in their bodies, despite feeling sexual excitement in their minds.

Arousal during rape is one of the clearest instances of sexual discordance. Despite feelings of horror and attempts to deter the offender, it can be quite common for women to experience a genital response during rape. Evolutionary psychologists speculate that this automatic response may have evolved to protect the woman from infections or trauma to the vagina and other reproductive areas during sex. Unfortunately, the presence of vaginal lubrication (or even orgasm in some cases of women who have been raped) has been used completely inappropriately in court proceedings to indicate that the victim "must have wanted it, or else her body would not have become physically aroused." This is a disturbing and wrong conclusion to draw and one that is not at all supported by science. If lawyers and judges had a better understanding of sexual discordance in women, such preposterous claims would not be made. Women's bodies and their minds may tell different stories about sexual arousal, but as Kate Harding points out in her book *Asking for It: The Alarming Rise of Rape Culture and What We Can Do About It*, it is a woman's mouth that should be listened to. A woman's self-report of how she feels is the ultimate reporter of her experience and the only way that consent can be given.

At the opposite pole of sexual discordance is sexual concordance—when there is agreement between mental and physical sexual arousal. This is a situation when a woman experiences physical sexual arousal and a parallel increase in mental sexual arousal. The two types of arousal increase to (roughly) the same degree. Concordance—and discordance, for that matter—is not simply a matter of whether arousal is present or absent, but is also a matter of degree. Figure 3 shows the change in self-reported mental and physical arousal in women who switched from watching a neutral (nonsexual) film to an erotic film.

High sexual concordance occurs when the amount of mental sexual arousal corresponds to a very similar degree to the increase in physical sexual arousal, as shown in Graph A. Low sexual concordance, on the other hand, takes place when both mental and physical sexual arousal increase (in response to an erotic stimulus), but to different levels, as shown in Graph B. In other words, the women whose responses are shown in Graph B found that their body was sexually aroused but their mind was not.

Although much of what we know about how the mind and the body respond to sexual triggers comes from sophisticated and methodical laboratory studies at universities and research centers in hospitals—and this approach might be criticized for not mimicking the natural environment of a person's home—it turns out that measuring sexual response in a private research laboratory at a university or hospital provides an even better window into a participant's sexual functioning at home. There are several reasons for this. First, the environment in a private research lab is free of distractions typically found at home (for example, ringing telephones, baskets of laundry, the threat of someone walking in). Second, the sexual stimuli used in laboratories (typically an erotic film or narrated fantasy or sexual images) have been previously tested on others and found to elicit a sexual response. And third, the tools used to measure physical sexual arousal are safe and specific to sexual arousal, and they allow researchers to draw conclusions about different facets of sexual arousal.

Figure 3. Possible relationship between self-reported arousal and genital arousal in women. The top graph represents close agreement between self-reported arousal and the body's sexual arousal as women watch an erotic film. The bottom graph represents a physical sexual response but a neutral mental response, or lack of agreement.

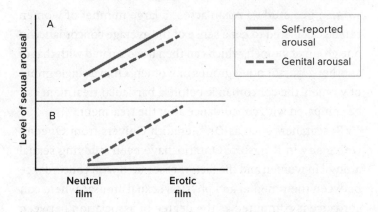

Relationship between self-reported and genital sexual arousal while women view neutral and erotic films

In the case of natal women (women born with female genital structures), much of the research identifying women who have low levels of sexual concordance has been based on measurements of physical genital response with the vaginal photoplethysmograph (which we discussed earlier). The probe is a safe, sterile tampon-shaped device that women insert into their own vagina. Once in place, it cannot be felt, just as tampons aren't felt. The participating women sit back comfortably on a reclining chair and watch neutral and erotic films, while the probe detects moment-by-moment changes in vaginal blood flow that are thought to provide an indirect measure of physical sexual response. At the same time, the women use a hand-held lever or computer mouse (known to those of us in the lab as the "arousometer") to indicate their current level of sexual arousal. As they are watching the film, they can move the lever or mouse to correspond to their current level of mental sexual arousal. As they feel more turned on, they push the lever or the mouse forward, and as their sexual interest lessens, they pull back on it. Scientists then use statistics to estimate a woman's concordance between physical sexual response and self-reported arousal. Once this estimate is derived for each woman in a study, a mean across a large number of women can be calculated to get a sense of the average concordance in one group of women, which can then be compared with that of another group or other groups of women. Or in a single group of women, the concordance before a particular treatment can be compared with concordance after the treatment.

Researchers such as Dr. Meredith Chivers from Queen's University in Kingston, Ontario, have been studying sexual arousal in women and the factors associated with concordance between their mental and physical sexual arousal, where concordance is computed as the degree of association between the probe's and the lever's ratings. Chivers's research indicates that the average correlation between women's physical sexual arousal response and their mental sexual arousal is about +0.26. (A correlation of +1.0 would indicate perfect positive agreement between mental and physical arousal, or complete concordance, and a correlation of -1.0 would indicate perfect negative agreement, or complete discordance. A number close to zero would indicate no relationship between those facets of arousal.) A concordance estimate of +0.26 indicates a low level of agreement between genital and mental sexual arousal when women are exposed to sexually arousing material. In other words, one aspect of their arousal is increasing more markedly than the other.

Chivers's research shows that the age of a woman, her relationship status, and whether or not she has a sexual dysfunction do not seem to alter this low degree of association between mental and physical arousal. In men, however, the level of sexual concordance is much higher, at about +0.66, indicating that as men's physical sexual arousal increases in response to a sexual stimulus, there is a closer corresponding increase in their level of self-reported arousal, or feeling turned on. In other words, their minds and bodies become aroused synchronously when they are exposed to sexually explicit material. Moreover, concordance tends to increase as men age, suggesting, perhaps, that learning may have a role to play in men's greater alignment of physical and mental sexual arousal.

HOW IS CONCORDANCE
RELATED TO MINDFULNESS?

CAN MINDFULNESS AFFECT concordance? To understand this, let's consider another woman's story.

Gianna is an otherwise physically healthy woman who sought treatment for a lack of sexual response and a very low level of sexual desire. When she viewed a sexually explicit, female-friendly film in our research laboratory, she moved the hand-held "arousometer" only one notch forward, corresponding to a very low level of feeling turned on while watching the attractive actors kissing, petting, and eventually having sex. As she watched the male actor please his female partner, first with a sensual foot massage and then with a very generous helping of oral sex, she looked down at her watch to see how much longer the testing would take. She told us afterward that she started making a mental grocery list, planning her kids' birthday party, and reminding herself to phone her mother. It was not that Gianna was turned off but rather that she felt indifferent to what she was watching. She also disliked "the look" of the female actress—too blonde, too thin, and too pretty.

Yet, the probe registered something very different. In the next room, the researchers saw evidence of a very strong increase in genital sexual response within about a minute of the erotic film's appearance on the large flat-screen TV in the adjacent testing room. When the researchers debriefed with Gianna at the end of the testing session and asked her if she had any emotional reactions to the film, she said that it was "Meh, kind of OK, I guess." Not surprisingly, her sexual concordance was very low (about +0.15), reflecting the fact that her body was aroused but her mind was not.

Gianna then took part in eight weekly sessions of mindfulness-based group treatment. By learning to pay attention to sensations within her body, she realized that she was completely distracted during sex. Even when she noticed a physical sexual response in her body, she rarely focused on it and instead got lost in an array of thoughts about planning for various events. It was not that sex was unpleasant or unpleasurable for her—when she tuned in, she reported finding it very pleasurable. She believed that as long as her body was going through the "motions" of sex, she should be able to have an orgasm. For her, it was irrelevant where her mind was. In our treatment, we targeted this misconception and explained the importance of reciprocal communication between the mind and the body. We conveyed to Gianna that a satisfying sexual response was not a reflex and that two-way communication between her brain and her body was essential for her sexual response. We also explained that distractions can impede this communication and that mindfulness was intended to strengthen it. We anchored her experience to Basson's circular sexual response cycle (see Figure 1 in Chapter 4), emphasizing that using mindfulness skills to tune in to her physical arousal might elicit sexual desire, which would then further increase her motivation for the sex she was having. Gianna completely related to this conceptualization of low sexual motivation and came to believe that what she focused on during sex was under her control, rather than in control of her. She also readily identified with the model of responsive sexual desire in which her sexual arousal came first and desire emerged after.

However, Gianna struggled to incorporate mindfulness into her life because the very preoccupations that kept her busy and distracted during sex also interfered with her commitment to complete the daily mindfulness exercises. With an hour-long commute book-ending a nine-hour work day, followed by exercise, community volunteer work, and household chores, Gianna had no time to sit on a meditation cushion and pay attention to her breath for thirty minutes. Yet, week after week, she attended the group mindfulness sessions, took part in forty-minute mindfulness meditations led by the instructor, and claimed how much she enjoyed the practices and wished that she could incorporate them into her daily life. However, during an extended mindfulness practice one day, Gianna said, through tears, "I just don't get it! I can be so present in my body when I'm here in this isolated room with a group of strangers, and yet at home, when I try to be with my physical sensations in my comfortable and familiar environment, I feel like I get even more distracted, and I just don't feel anything in my body!"

We now have scientific evidence from our research that women who adopt a regular mindfulness practice experience increased concordance between genital response and mental sexual arousal. When we looked closer at the data, we observed that the women became more aware of their physical sexual arousal, and this drove the greater concordance between their mental and physical arousal. In Gianna's case, after the eight weeks of daily practice, which sometimes only lasted ten minutes because of time pressures, her concordance level in the laboratory increased to a higher degree of concordance between physical and mental arousal.

We have also found that mindfulness improves this mind-body sexual communication significantly more than other effective psychological treatments, such as cognitive behavioral therapy (CBT), which is not aimed explicitly at bringing awareness to the body's sensations. As you'll recall from Chapter 2, CBT involves teaching women relaxation exercises and using cognitive challenging techniques to replace negative thoughts with more balanced ways of thinking. Childhood sexual abuse can have a devastating impact on a woman's sexuality, and some women continue to struggle during sex even if they are in a happy, satisfying, and safe relationship where sex is only ever consensual. As a result of previous sexual trauma, some women continue to dissociate during sex to protect themselves both physically and emotionally, as they learned to do during the abuse.

Dissociation can continue later in the woman's life, when she is in a safe and consensual encounter, because the brain has "learned" to dissociate in response to sexual triggers. What a distressing situation these women find themselves in when years after the abuse—and for many even after years of counseling to address the aftermath of the abuse—they experience these difficulties with sex.

We have found that mindfulness can be a useful tool for women with a history of sexual trauma as children who now as adults experience high levels of sex-related distress and dissociate in response to sexual triggers. In our research, we invited half of the women to take part in group mindfulness sessions and assigned the other half to a CBT group, where they essentially learned to identify and change negative thoughts related to sexuality. Although both groups experienced significant improvements in sex-related distress, the women who learned mindfulness experienced a greater increase in their genital-subjective concordance than women in the other treatment group. In other words, following mindfulness training, the women's self-reporting of sexual arousal corresponded more closely with their body's sexual arousal; their mental and physical sexual arousal were more in sync with one another.

INTEROCEPTIVE AWARENESS

ALTHOUGH WE HAVE evidence only from a few research studies to support our suggestion that improved sexual arousal concordance occurs after women practice mindfulness, a larger body of research shows the effects of mindfulness on other types of mind-body concordance. One of these is *interoception*, which refers to a person's ability to detect their own internal bodily sensations. There is great variability in people's awareness levels of their bodies. For example, some people are aware of their heart rate and can estimate, within a few beats of accuracy, their own heartbeats per minute. Other people are aware of small changes in muscle tension and can use that awareness by employing a muscle relaxation strategy to prevent harmful increases in muscle tension. Some women can sense when they ovulate.

All of us lie somewhere on the spectrum of being interoceptively aware, with some people being highly aware and others highly unaware, and most people being somewhere in between. There is also evidence that judgmental thoughts about being inadequate or feelings of embarrassment, guilt, or anxiety can interfere with a person's interoceptive awareness. The good news is that interoceptive awareness can be cultivated with training.

But why would we want to increase our interoceptive awareness? Is being aware of your heart rate really that important? We know that people who tend to focus more on the external features of their body also tend to have lower interoceptive awareness. Some early theorists believed that attention could not be equally allocated to one's external appearance and to internal signals produced by the body. But research has more recently shown that women who are low in interoceptive awareness and self-objectify their bodies more than men tend to have more clinical symptoms of such conditions as depression and disordered eating. Researchers have also found that having low awareness of the internal body may lead women to objectify the external aspects of their body more and have reasoned that teaching women to be more aware of their internal bodily activities may decrease their objectification of their own bodies. This awareness may even be useful for women who tend to worry about what their bodies look like during sex, as they will be focusing instead on what is happening inside their body.

And it turns out that women can improve their interoceptive awareness. People with experience in Vipassana meditation tend to have much more visceral awareness of their body than professional dancers, for example, who are aware of their external body but not necessarily their internal body sensations, and both of these groups have more body awareness than nondancers and nonmeditators.

In one study done at the University of California, Berkeley, in 2010, meditators, dancers, and a control group who neither meditated nor danced were shown short funny, violent, and neutral films. As they watched a variety of emotional films, such as a comedy, a horror film, films depicting disgusting images, and a sad film, they had to use a dial to indicate the emotional intensity they felt in reaction to the films. At the same time, their heart rate was measured with sensors and a polygraph, and this was correlated with the participants' self-reports of emotional intensity to come up with a measure of concordance. The results showed that the meditators had the highest degree of concordance between their body's reactions and their emotional reactions to the films. The dancers had a slightly lower degree of mind-body concordance, and the control group had the lowest degree of concordance.

This study could be interpreted to mean that with training in attending to the internal sensations of the body, it is possible to develop greater alignment of one's self-reported emotions and one's physiological reaction to emotional events or scenes. Thus, someone who has had mindfulness training and whose heart rate increases while watching a frightening film is more likely to have a corresponding increase in their reports of feeling scared or anxious than someone who has not had mindfulness training. The researchers concluded that those who are trained to develop increased attention to and awareness of their internal body sensations have access to more accurate information about the state of their bodies, and this may lead them to have increased positive affect, or emotions, and better overall well-being.

One of the ways that mindfulness significantly increases interoceptive awareness is through altering brain activity. In a study from the University of Toronto comparing novice meditators with experienced meditators, participants had areas of their brain scanned with functional magnetic resonance imaging (fMRI) under two different conditions. In one condition, the participants were given instructions to focus mindfully on their moment-by-moment sensations and during moments of distraction to gently guide their attention back to the present moment (this was called the "experiential focus" condition). In the other condition, the participants were presented with words and told to figure out what a presented word meant for them, to judge themselves for what they were feeling, and to allow themselves to get caught up in the contents of their thoughts (this was called the "narrative focus" condition). There were distinct differences in brain activation when participants engaged in mindfulness and when they allowed themselves to get caught up in their thoughts. Mindfulness was associated with less brain activity along the cortical midline in the prefrontal cortex and in the amygdala, considered the emotion center of the brain.

There were other interesting findings from this study. The group that had participated in an eight-week mindfulness-based stress-reduction (MBSR) program showed reduced activity in areas of the brain associated with emotions, suggesting that one of the ways mindfulness is effective is through reducing emotional activation associated with body sensations. Thus, when one experiences the sensations of pain, for example, mindfulness reduces the tendency to feel emotions such as sadness, anger, and despair in response to that pain. Similarly, as meditators become more adept at recognizing changes in their body, they react less emotionally to those changes.

Furthermore, when meditators in this study were distracted, they maintained awareness of their body, whereas those untrained in mindfulness did not. The researchers postulated that even in stressful conditions, experienced meditators maintain an awareness of what is happening in their body at all times. And the more daily mindfulness that participants practiced, the more they could maintain this state of body awareness.

How might this be relevant to women with low sexual desire? It may be that meditation allows women to pay attention to sensations in their body and to have fewer negative emotional reactions to those sensations. For many women, signs of arousal can provoke anxiety, resentment, anger, or other negative emotions, and the presence of these emotions may directly impede continued arousal and, of course, sexual desire. Perhaps mindfulness allows women to tune in to the body without eliciting strong negative and potentially distracting emotions. Or if those negative feelings do occur, perhaps mindfulness skills help women to notice them in a more distanced way, without reacting to them. To date, almost no research has focused on women with sex-related concerns, like Gianna, and whether mindfulness improves sexual desire and sexual concordance by targeting interoceptive awareness. Unfortunately, research into this question is in its infancy.

In our own research at the University of British Columbia, groups of women with low desire are exposed to eight weeks of mindfulness practice and fill out a questionnaire before and after the training so that we can measure whether they experience any changes in their interoceptive awareness. The questionnaire includes such statements as "I notice changes in my breathing, such as whether it slows down or speeds up" and "I can maintain awareness of my inner bodily sensations even when there is a lot going on around me," and we compare their levels on each of these questions from baseline to after completion of the eight-week mindfulness program. We found that after the eight weeks, the women had significant improvements in four key aspects of interoceptive awareness: the tendency to not ignore or distract themselves from uncomfortable sensations, the ability to sustain and control attention to their bodily sensations, the ability to regulate their own distress by paying attention to their bodily sensations, and the ability to actively listen to their bodies.

In addition to each of these improvements in interoceptive awareness, the women with low sexual desire also experienced significant improvements in levels of depression and rumination (the tendency to think about things over and over), and how quickly they became anxious. As the women became more aware of their internal bodily sensations over the eight weeks of the group sessions, they experienced more sexual desire and less sex-related distress. The findings related to improved interoceptive awareness suggest that staying present, paying attention to the present moment, and listening to one's body may be key for helping women with low sexual desire.

In a 2011 study of college students at Brown University, half of the participants participated in a mindfulness program while the others attended a religious studies course. After the training, participants viewed a series of sexual and nonsexual photos, and the time it took them to rate their perceived physical arousal (a measure of interoception) was recorded. The researchers found that at the start of the study, the women took significantly longer than men to notice and rate their own physical sexual arousal. The slower reaction times to sexual photos were associated with the women's higher ratings of depression, anxiety, and self-judgment—which are known to directly affect sexual functioning. However, mindfulness led to a significantly faster "reaction time," meaning that the women could take note of and rate their own physical responses more quickly after practicing mindfulness. I found it interesting that this faster reaction time was specific to the sexual photos only, indicating that the improvements in interoceptive awareness were specific to sexually arousing photos. Furthermore, their improved interoceptive awareness was directly related to less self-judgment and anxiety and higher self-acceptance and general well-being. As they became more aware of their internal bodily sensations, they were not as hard on themselves, experienced less anxiety, and had an improved overall outlook on life.

The findings from this study suggest that negative mood and self-judgment can interfere with women's interoceptive ability and that this can further impede sexual response when women are faced with erotic triggers. Mindfulness directly targets this problem. After mindfulness training, the women in the study became faster at tuning in to their bodies and could differentiate between different sensations in their bodies—and did both with less self-judgment and more self-acceptance. Although it was not clear from the findings whether mindfulness caused the psychological changes or whether the improvements in psychological domains led women to be more mindful, the researchers suspected that mindfulness was responsible for the effects by removing the psychological barriers, which allowed the women to tune in to their body's sensations.

So what can we conclude about the effects of mindfulness training on internal body awareness, and how might this information help women who experience low sexual desire? The research shows that women low in interoceptive awareness are more likely to have clinical symptoms such as depression, poor self-image, and symptoms of an eating disorder, and training in mindfulness improves each of these conditions. Women with little interoceptive awareness are also more likely to judge themselves negatively, which impedes sexual desire. Furthermore, we have evidence that, in general, women's concordance between their self-reported and physical sexual response is low, and that training in mindfulness significantly increases the degree of mind-to-body communication and improves self-reported interoceptive awareness. In turn, improvements in women's interoceptive awareness predict improvements in their levels of sexual desire and reductions in their feelings of sex-related distress.

The take-home message is this: mindfulness teaches women to become more aware of their internal bodily sensations, including sexual sensations, and this may improve their motivations for sex and increase their tendency to notice sexual arousal and have that arousal trigger sexual desire.

Could it really be this simple—that teaching women to tune in to their body, to the signs that their body is already producing, and making them aware of these sensations can be enough to trigger sexual desire? I offer a tentative "yes" to this question. Why tentative? Because awareness of internal bodily sensations is only one of potentially many different ways that mindfulness exerts its beneficial effects on sexual desire. Without a doubt, when we pay attention to the body in a kind, compassionate, nonjudgmental, and present-oriented way, it offers us a new way of being in the world. And that new way of being might just be critical for the sexual satisfaction that so many women crave.

CHAPTER 7

IF YOU'RE HAPPY AND YOU KNOW IT

———————

Sex is always about emotions. Good sex is about free emotions;
bad sex is about blocked emotions.

DEEPAK CHOPRA via purplebuddhaproject.tumblr.com

ACH OF US has felt sad at some point in our lives. You may experience sadness as feeling down, depressed, and lethargic. Those around you may see a frown or tear-drenched eyes or a downcast gaze. But for approximately 7 percent of the U.S. population over any single year, this sadness can be extreme, can last for weeks with no letting up, and can interfere with a person's ability to participate in the events of their life.

Over the course of a person's lifetime, there is on average a 15 percent chance of developing depression, with women having a higher likelihood than men. Extreme and lasting sadness is formally referred to as a major depressive episode and is diagnosed when someone feels depressed or has lost interest in activities that were formerly enjoyable, a condition known as anhedonia. Other symptoms include weight loss or gain, difficulties with sleep (either too much or insomnia), fatigue or loss of energy, a feeling of slowness or sluggishness, feelings of worthlessness or guilt, difficulties concentrating or making decisions, and thoughts of death. Some people may also make an elaborate suicide plan or even attempt to commit suicide. During a depressive episode, it is common to experience at least five of these symptoms almost all day, on most days, over a two-week period. For some people, this constellation of symptoms can continue for many weeks or months.

Depression is much more common in women than in men. Several theories have been put forward to account for this disparity. Biological factors, such as women's greater genetic predisposition to depression and variations in hormone levels as a result of the menstrual cycle, pregnancy, childbirth, and menopause may account for women's higher risk of developing depression. Another finding is that women are predisposed to depression because they tend to ruminate over past events more than men do. They are also more negatively affected than men by relationship distress or conflict. One of the most potent psychological explanations, however, is that women are more prone to stress than men, and repeated chronic stress can act as a trigger for depression. The higher rates of depression in women may also be a by-product of the fact that they live longer than men or that they are more likely than men to seek help for depression and therefore benefit from having a diagnosis. And while it could be argued that men may have high rates of depression also but are less likely than women to ask for help and therefore less likely to be diagnosed, the experts remain convinced that depression rates are higher in women than in men.

DEPRESSION AND LOW SEXUAL DESIRE

ONE OF THE hallmarks of a depressive episode is apathy. A depressed person may have lost interest in activities they previously enjoyed, such as dancing, cooking, bowling, or socializing in general. They may also have lost interest in sex, even if they previously enjoyed it and initiated it.

Take Sheila as an example. She had always enjoyed sex. By the age of fifty-two she had had three long-term relationships and several short-term relationships, and in each of them she would both initiate sexual activity and be receptive when her partner initiated sex. During the early stages of physical contact, she experienced many of the classic signs of arousal, such as increases in skin sensitivity, vaginal throbbing, and lubrication, and these sensations reliably intensified as she engaged in sex. Most of her sexual encounters had been with women, though she occasionally had sex with men, which led to similar positive sexual feelings of pleasure and satisfaction.

However, over a span of fourteen months, Sheila lost both her parents to chronic medical illnesses, a reorganization at work left her unemployed, and her best friend moved to another state. The grief she experienced in reaction to these major life events triggered a period of intense sadness, which culminated in a full-blown major depressive episode. Her diagnosis was confirmed by her primary care provider, who suggested that she consider a selective serotonin reuptake inhibitor (SSRI), a class of antidepressant medications, to help her cope during this period of grief, loss, and transition. She agreed.

Although Sheila had been on the antidepressant for twelve weeks, her mood had not returned to normal. She had pulled away from her friends and family, had stopped socializing, and was spending most of her waking hours in front of the television. However, she missed having sex and told herself that she should muster up the motivation to have sex given that it had always been a reliable mood enhancer for her. Sheila had a few acquaintances with whom she used to regularly engage in friends-with-benefits sex, and she thought she could jump-start her mood by having a satisfying orgasm. She was sorely disappointed, however. Although she and one partner engaged in the same sexual acts that in the past had regularly and reliably been exciting, sex now felt, in her words, "like a tiny gray blip on a previously multicolor full-sexual screen." In sexual encounters with other casual partners, Sheila lied, telling them, "That was great; thanks for boosting my mood"; yet inside she still felt miserable and apathetic. Acknowledging that what used to provide so much joy and pleasure for her had now lost its potency left Sheila feeling even more depressed. She was clearly caught in a vicious cycle of depression, as depicted in Figure 4.

Figure 4. The vicious cycle of depression, apathy, and low sexual desire

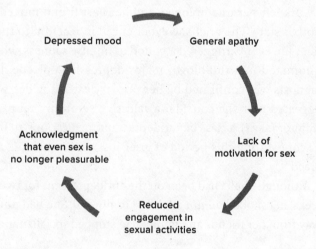

Depressed mood

General apathy

Lack of motivation for sex

Reduced engagement in sexual activities

Acknowledgment that even sex is no longer pleasurable

Clinicians have long been aware of the strong association between depression and sexuality. Large studies find that at least three-quarters of patients seeking treatment for depression experience low sexual desire, and although they may also have other sexual concerns, the loss of libido seems to be the most prevalent. Although for many people antidepressants are an effective treatment for depression, for many others they can also worsen the sexual symptoms and further dampen mood. The link between depression and sex is complicated by the fact that people with depression are also at a higher risk of having other medical disorders, such as diabetes or cardiovascular disease, and these conditions also negatively affect sexual functioning.

Does the depression cause the loss of sexual desire, or does low sexual motivation lead people to be depressed? This is an interesting question that has been explored in many different research studies. In Sheila's case, her depression was due to a series of significant stressors and losses, and the depression caused her sexual problems. However, as the unfulfilling and frustrating sexual encounters continued, Sheila's mood slipped more and more. For Sheila, and for many others, there is a bidirectional relationship between depression and low sexual desire, as is depicted in Figure 4, with low mood leading to loss of sexual desire, which in turn further triggers depression. In a meta-analysis review of several large studies exploring the relationship between depression and sex, those with depression had a 50 to 70 percent increased risk of developing sexual dysfunction, and those with sexual dysfunction had a 130 to 210 percent increased risk of developing depression. Sexual difficulties following depression can lead to withdrawal from one's usual social life and activities, performance anxiety during sex, and sexual aversion. And all of these can further drive mood into a downward spiral.

Although there are many symptoms of depression, researchers have found that anhedonia is most strongly linked to depression, and it is more strongly associated with depression than anxiety is. In a 2014 study in which women kept a daily record of their mood, anxiety, and level of sexual desire, researchers found that the intensity of a woman's anhedonia on one day predicted her level of sexual desire the next day. These findings led the researchers to question the previously held belief that there was a direct link between depression and sexual desire—that either low mood led to loss of desire or lack of interest in sex led to a worsening of mood. These researchers postulated that the relationship between depression and low desire is somewhat more complex, that an underlying factor may lead to both the depression and the loss of sexual desire.

There is much that researchers still do not know about the brain-related changes that might explain the link between depression and loss of interest in sex, but it is possible that alterations in the brain's dopamine system might be responsible for both the apathy and low libido. This link has spurred interest in an entire field of research looking at the effectiveness of dopamine-acting drugs in improving women's sexual desire. Chapter 2 mentions Addyi (flibanserin), which has dopamine-enhancing effects on the brain but is not without its limitations. The fact that Addyi cannot be mixed with alcohol due to their combined effects of excessive drowsiness and a drop in blood pressure is a serious concern for many women. Hopefully, future medications will not impose this limitation.

DEPRESSION AND MENOPAUSE

IN ADDITION TO apathy, depression is characterized by strong automatic thoughts such as "Things will never get better" or "No matter what I do, I'm a failure." Beliefs such as these are especially prominent among middle-aged women, and this population seems to be particularly vulnerable to both depression and low sexual function. There is evidence that approximately half of women attending a menopause clinic are currently experiencing depression and other negative psychological symptoms, such as irritability, anxiety, and feeling exhausted, and that these are associated with poor sexual functioning as women go through menopause.

The perimenopause is a time of social and personal change for many women. Hormonally, it is defined as the cessation of ovarian function and a sharp decline in the production of estrogen from the ovaries. Levels of follicle-stimulating hormone (FSH) from the brain increase, and levels of testosterone remain relatively consistent (though there is an overall decline in testosterone levels over a woman's lifespan). During the menopausal transition (which can last for many months or even years), many women experience physical changes such as hot flushes, sleep disturbances, night sweats, thinning of the vaginal wall and vaginal dryness, and mood changes. The decrease in vaginal elasticity and increase in vaginal dryness can lead to dyspareunia (pain from vaginal penetration) for many women, and as you can likely imagine, the repeated experience of pain through vaginal intercourse can lead a woman to very quickly lose her interest in intercourse.

Surgical menopause takes place when the ovaries are removed, a procedure known as bilateral salpingo-oophorectomy. Bilateral salpingo-oophorectomy is often performed at the same time as a hysterectomy (removal of the uterus), a procedure that as many as one in five women will undergo by the age of fifty-five. Much of the science exploring the effects of bilateral salpingo-oophorectomy on sexual functioning has been mixed, with some studies showing a definitive link between removal of the ovaries and loss of sexual desire, and other studies showing no relationship.

A 2008 Australian study compared women aged forty-five to sixty-five who underwent natural menopause, defined as having at least one full year without menstruation, with women in the same age range who underwent surgical menopause and followed both groups a year into their post-menopausal period. Women in the two groups were similar in terms of duration of their relationships, education, income, body mass index, and duration of menopause. Sexual desire, arousal, frequency of sex, and orgasm did not differ between the two groups. The only variable related to sexual function that differed between them was vaginal lubrication—with the surgical menopause group reporting twice the frequency of "no lubrication" as those who had gone through natural menopause.

The researchers interpreted the findings to mean that nonhormonal factors contribute more to sexual desire than hormonal factors do, except in the case of vaginal lubrication, which is largely determined by estrogens produced in the ovaries. A much larger prospective study of women who received a bilateral salpingo-oophorectomy for benign reasons (for example, bleeding disorders) found no differences between the hysterectomy alone and hysterectomy plus bilateral salpingo-oophorectomy group on any measure of sexual functioning or psychological well-being a year after surgery.

The indications for a bilateral salpingo-oophorectomy

vary, ranging from treatment of fibroids and endometriosis to the presence of a gynecologic cancer or even prophylactic treatment among women who are gene carriers for breast or ovarian cancer. The women in the study described above who underwent surgical menopause elected to have their ovaries removed, and this may have affected their sexuality in a *positive way*. It seems that young women who have their ovaries removed have a much more marked decline in desire for sex than women who have their ovaries removed when they are older. One interpretation of this phenomenon is that younger women may mourn the loss of fertility or fear the effects of rapid aging that come with bilateral salpingo-oophorectomy more than older women do.

Clearly, the effects of the perimenopause and postmenopause on sexual functioning involve a complex interplay of hormonal, psychological, and social factors. For example, the changing roles at home and at work, the "empty nest" effect or even grown children returning home (and the stress associated with that), and changes in employment can affect different women quite differently. Menopausal symptoms that interfere with sleep and can trigger fatigue, declining health, loss of reproductive ability, and negative attitudes about aging all have a potent effect on mood as well as sexuality. Some women fiercely oppose the aging process and will go to great lengths to stall or prevent its negative effects. Interestingly, women who have a more negative attitude toward menopause tend to have more menopausal symptoms than women who have a more positive attitude. Furthermore, attitudes about aging and feelings about a partner were found to outweigh the effects of changing hormone levels on the sexual functioning of menopausal women. Beliefs trump biology.

MINDFULNESS AS A
TREATMENT FOR DEPRESSION

RETURNING TO DEPRESSION, there are enormous individual differences across women in the symptoms and duration of depression, and its impact on other aspects of their life. Also, not all aspects of sexual functioning are impaired when a woman experiences depression in midlife. In fact, one large study of American women from across the United States in 2004 found that middle-aged depressed women had a higher frequency of masturbation than middle-aged women who were not depressed. How can depression lead some women to masturbate *more*? It is likely that for this group of women, masturbation serves as a self-soothing activity that offers a temporary state of pleasure in the context of reduced sexual pleasure with a partner and general anhedonia.

Sheila's experience illustrated this phenomenon. Although she was depressed and apathetic toward sex, she masturbated to feel pleasure and to remind herself of her former capacity for a sexual response that did not depend on a partner or on managing their expectations. A similar phenomenon occurs in men, particularly gay men, where masturbation is often identified as a method of dealing with stress and anxiety.

Mindfulness has long been used to treat depression and was the subject of a vast number of scientific studies long before it was ever systematically applied to the treatment of sexual concerns. For this reason, it is the ideal treatment for women whose depression contributes to a loss of desire and whose diminishing libido further dampens mood. Mindfulness-based cognitive therapy (MBCT) (discussed in Chapter 3) was developed specifically to prevent people who had a history of depressive episodes from experiencing a depressive relapse or falling into another depression in the future. Mindfulness is more effective at reducing symptoms of depression and at keeping depressive symptoms at bay than either education alone or simply providing a supportive environment where people can talk and share their feelings.

How does mindfulness reduce symptoms of depression? Mindfulness does not make a depressed person ignore their sadness or rid the mind of sad and ruminative thoughts, but it does lessen the negative effects of long-term depression so that a depressed person can take action as soon as they notice the early signs of depression.

As previously mentioned, mindfulness has two key aspects: awareness of sensations (including body and breath sensations as well as sounds and thoughts) and adoption of a nonjudgmental attitude toward whatever one notices during that period of awareness. During a mindfulness practice, a person uses their attentional resources to continually redirect their focus onto their present sensations (whether those are breath, body, sound, or thought sensations), and as they do so, they continue to observe their sensations with a greater degree of acuity. Then they invite an accepting attitude toward those physical or mental sensations by not judging them—or themselves for having those sensations. This allows them to steer away from their typical ruminating, worrying, and judging thought patterns. If they feel sad, instead of getting caught up in the story behind their sadness, they would focus on their bodily sensations associated with sadness: "I notice a flutter in my belly. I sense a depth and intensity to my breathing. I feel a tension in my right lower back. My heart feels like it is beating quickly," instead of "Why does this always happen to me! Will I ever get out of this deep, dark place? Am I destined to feel this horribly forever?"

The thirteenth-century Persian poet Mewlana Jalaluddin Rumi explored the concept of an accepting approach to emotions in his poem "The Guest House,"* which characterizes emotions as "unexpected visitors" and encourages us to treat all emotions that arrive at the door—the positive as well as the negative—as welcome guests. In telling us to be "grateful for whoever comes," Rumi believes that even sadness is valuable and may teach us something. "The Guest House" also encourages us to treat all emotions equally ("Welcome and entertain them all!"), which may be a way of responding nonjudgmentally to unpleasant emotions.

By practicing mindfulness, you learn to observe and accept your feelings, reduce the tendency to ruminate about them, and experience mindfulness as a form of coping with them. Mindfulness does not prevent those emotions from arising—or, using the analogy of "The Guest House," you do not turn away those unpleasant emotions when they knock at your door. Rather, mindfulness may allow you to identify and observe those emotions earlier, before they become intense and destructive.

A systematic review of the evidence evaluating mindfulness for preventing a relapse in depression found that it was especially effective for people who have had three or more previous depressive episodes, and also that the degree of improvement was not related to how much mindfulness was practiced at home.

Mindfulness-based cognitive therapy for preventing depressive relapse involves teaching participants to "turn toward" their bodily sensations and to practice accepting the

---

* *Rumi, J. (1997). The essential Rumi (C. Banks, Trans.). Edison, NJ: Castle Books,* p. 109.

sensations as they appear. Participants are also encouraged to notice their negative emotions and to accept them. The participants practice relating to negative thoughts and ruminations as habits of the mind and to detach from their content. In the mindfulness groups we run at the University of British Columbia, we often put our own spin on Jon Kabat-Zinn's advice and encourage women to view negative thoughts as being about as important as what they ate for breakfast last week.

It is likely that the improvements in clinical symptoms of depression directly correspond to changes in the brain that occur as a result of mindfulness practice. For example, mindfulness practice leads to less activation in the emotion center in the brain, the amygdala, while increasing activity in the part of the brain that is responsible for cultivating awareness of bodily cues (as discussed in Chapter 6). If you are able to notice and accept the initial feeling of depression as soon as it starts, you may be better equipped to engage in a helpful behavior—such as exercise or calling a friend—that could minimize the negative consequences of a full-blown depression.

In one of our earliest studies of mindfulness for women with sexual dysfunction related to treatment for gynecologic cancer, most women entering the study had a mild level of depression, and their symptoms were highly correlated with sex-related distress. The more depressed the women were, the more distress about their sexual difficulties they had. Although all of the women experienced a significant improvement in their depression with only three monthly sessions of mindfulness-based therapy (and daily mindfulness practice at home), those women who initially had higher levels of depression appeared to benefit the most. Furthermore, the women who were among the more depressed at the beginning reported a greater improvement in their experience of pleasure in response to genital stimulation. In other words, it seemed that the mindfulness-based therapy improved not only their mood but also the women's feelings of physical pleasure, and both of these effects were more pronounced among the women who were initially more depressed.

In 2008 we completed a study evaluating group mindfulness for women seeking treatment for low sexual desire, and found that women in the study who had a history of sexual abuse tended to have greater improvements in mood than women without a history of sexual abuse. It is possible that the effects of our intervention, which again was originally developed to specifically target sexual symptoms, are most potent among women who have more symptoms to begin with.

Depression and anxiety have long been known to negatively affect sexual functioning, but they also interfere with a woman's interoceptive awareness. Increases in depression (and anxiety) may serve as distractors, effectively blocking a woman's ability to notice internal bodily sensations. Another study, this one from Brown University in 2011, that evaluated the effects of mindfulness on interoceptive awareness found that after women participated in mindfulness training, they had faster reaction times to sexual images, which was associated with better interoceptive awareness and with improved psychological symptoms. Explained another way, as women practice mindfulness, their tendency to judge themselves negatively, ruminate, and become distracted is reduced, lessening their psychological distress and thus allowing them to react more quickly to sexual stimuli.

What happened to Sheila after she asked her family doctor if an antidepressant would improve her depression and her sexual desire? Luckily, Sheila's family doctor had participated in a program of mindfulness-based stress reduction (MBSR) for physicians and had benefited tremendously. She therefore recommended mindfulness to Sheila. After three months, Sheila had a significant improvement in her motivation for sex, and her mood improved to subclinical levels. She ruminated less about events of her life and no longer catastrophized when things did not go as planned. Like many patients who have benefited from a brief mindfulness-based program, Sheila was thrilled that she was feeling better in so many areas of her life.

HOW THE TREATMENT WORKS

AS RESEARCHERS, WE are interested not only in whether a given treatment works to resolve the difficulties faced by women like Sheila but also in *how* it works. The statistical technique known as "mediation analysis" allows us to examine whether the aspects of a person's experience we are trying to affect are indeed affected. Such analyses also help determine which aspects of treatment may be effective and which aspects may need to be improved.

Earlier we considered the role of attention when trying to understand how mindfulness works. Other studies, such as the work carried out at the University of Calgary along with the Tom Baker Cancer Centre, focused specifically on which aspects of a person's well-being might be responsible for the benefits that were seen to be gained with mindfulness. Researchers measured changes very soon after participants started to practice mindfulness and tracked these changes over the course of the two-month program to see which early changes might be most associated with greater improvements at the treatment's completion. They found that women's tendencies to attend to the present moment in a nonjudgmental manner were the earliest to change with treatment, whereas their learned ability to label emotions (without getting caught up in them) and to allow thoughts and feelings to come and go without ruminating about them were more likely to change later in the eight-week program. In other words, skills in paying attention, moment by moment, take hold early and predict overall improvements with a mindfulness-based approach, whereas skills in observing emotions and thoughts in a nonreactive and open manner take hold later in the treatment.

These research findings on the mediators of treatment effects help us to understand Sheila's experience more fully. In the first few weeks of practicing mindfulness, Sheila had a marked decrease in rumination and worry. These early changes likely directly contributed to Sheila's reduced tendency to judge herself later on, and that probably led to her improvements in many other aspects of mindfulness, such as observing and describing sensations in her body and in her mind. What we still do not know, however, is whether improvement in low mood earlier in treatment leads to later improvements in libido or whether there are more immediate improvements in desire with treatment that then predict later improvements in depression. This question will be answered in the next few years as research directly addressing this topic continues to emerge.

In my clinical practice, I now consistently recommend mindfulness-based therapy to women with low sexual desire who also struggle with depression or low mood. If this condition applies to you, you might consider closing your eyes at the end of this sentence, focusing on your internal bodily sensations, moment by moment, and taking the first step toward cultivating sexual desire and loosening the grip of depression.

BELIEVING IS EVERYTHING

YOU ARE PROBABLY familiar with the saying "Fake it till you make it." The truth of this statement, which highlights the impact of our attitudes on our behavior, has been demonstrated over and over as it applies to sexuality. Specifically, several large studies that have tracked women's sexual desire, behavior, mood, attitudes, and hormones over twenty years have found that women's beliefs about their sexuality outweigh the contribution of hormones to their level of sexual desire. For example, women who believe that they will continue to be sexually active with old age are more likely to have higher levels of sexual desire and behavior than women who do not believe this, regardless of their hormonal status. Laboratory research also finds that women who experimentally take on the mental image of being very sexually satisfied have a stronger physiological and mental sexual arousal response than women who do not adopt this frame of mind.

Researchers at the University of Washington, Seattle, carried out a study in which women with depression listened to an audiorecording of a woman's voice saying, "You enjoy your sexuality. You are confident with your own sexuality, and you feel comfortable asking for what you like sexually. You have a strong sense of who you are as a sexual woman." Later in the session they listened to a similar audiorecording that conveyed a negative message for them to adopt. After each of the recordings, the women watched a sexually explicit film while their physiological and mental sexual arousal levels were recorded. After listening to the positive audiorecording, the women had a greater level of positive feelings and lesser level of negative feelings than after listening to the negative audiorecording. After the positive recording, the women who were depressed also experienced a significant boost in their physiological sexual arousal, measured with the vaginal probe, as well as in their sense of mental sexual arousal.

The findings from this study have led us to create a similar exercise for our mindfulness-based groups at the University of British Columbia. After a dozen years of working with these groups, we have found that at least half of the participants have experienced depression in the past and that many of them currently experience some symptoms of depression. In our exercise, women are invited to "try on" a different sexual identity before taking part in a mindfulness practice. Through an exercise we call the pleasurable touch exercise, the women in our groups are asked to first imagine themselves as a sexually satisfied woman, someone who enjoys sexual touch and sexual behavior and who is happy with her sexual response. After some minutes of imagining this as their identity, they are guided to touch different parts of their body, including their genitals, in a mindfulness exercise. As with the experimental study discussed above, we predicted that adopting a positive sexual image would elicit positive feelings and decrease negative feelings in the moment, and we expected that the women could then become aware of these feelings during a subsequent mindfulness practice. The women participating in our mindfulness groups have told us that even when they did not believe their message to themselves about being a sexually satisfied woman, they could try that identity on during the exercise, and it allowed them to fully tune in to the sensations that arose as they engaged in touch. Here is the practice outlined in more detail. I invite you to try it.

Pleasurable Touch Exercise

Allow yourself approximately fifteen minutes for this exercise. You may also want to select a time when you feel better about yourself, when there are few distractions, and when you are unlikely to be interrupted. You may choose to have a water-based lubricant on hand for the genital touching parts of this exercise.

Read through the following instructions in their entirety before beginning the exercise. It is similar to the body awareness exercises that you have previously practiced. This one is goal-oriented, however, in that you will deliberately elicit and experience pleasurable body and genital sensations using touch. You will "try on" a sexual identity as you use touch, imagining that you are a sexual, sensual woman who enjoys her sexuality and is fully capable of a healthy sexual response. There is an important feedback loop from your genitals to your brain: as you notice sexual arousal in your body, your mind may interpret these sensations as being sexual, which then further increases the body's arousal.

1. Get into a comfortable position, perhaps lying down. Begin by closing your eyes and briefly checking in with how you feel in this moment. You might consider taking three minutes to first notice how your body feels overall, whether there are any particular emotions present, and whether your mind is particularly busy or not.

2. Next, focus your attention on the sense of touch or contact, starting with your feet. Notice the point at which your feet touch the surface beneath you, whether it is the bed or the floor. Focus attention on any sensations in your feet. Wiggle your toes and take note of what that feels like.

3. Move the focus of your attention up to your ankles, calves, and knees, noticing any sensations, tension, tingling, or feelings of warmth or cold there. Spend a few moments on each of these body parts as you move up your body.

4. Next, focus attention on your genitals. Imagine that you are sexy and fully capable of sexual response as you focus on this part of your body. Are you aware of any sensations in your labia, clitoris, or vagina? Notice if these sensations feel sexual. Contract your vaginal muscles and notice if that gives you a heightened sense of pleasure. Focus on the sensations produced in your genitals and take note of any thoughts or emotions that emerge. Remind yourself that these are the important parts when it comes to sexual pleasure and activity. They are yours.

5. Whenever you notice that you have forgotten about paying attention to the sensations in your genitals because your attention was focused on the content of a thought or story, congratulate yourself on becoming aware of that. Notice what your attention had been engaged with and then gently and kindly return your attention to the sensations in your genitals in this moment.

6. Next, move your hands to your genitals. While imagining to yourself that *you are a sexual, sensual woman,* lightly press your fingers on the area of your clitoris. Press on the area of your clitoral shaft and hood and then down each side of your outer labia. Lightly touch your inner labia. Feel the sensations produced by different amounts of pressure. Describe the sensations to yourself. Remind yourself that the goal of this exercise is to enhance your awareness of pleasurable sexual sensations. That is all.

7. Move your fingers down to touch the outer entrance of your vagina and then, when you are ready, guide one or

more fingers inside (use a water-based lubricant if you prefer). Describe the sensations to yourself. Contract the vaginal muscles and notice how it feels with your finger(s) inside. If you notice that you are caught up in *thinking about* the sensations or lack of sensations rather than experiencing the sensations themselves, gently and kindly redirect your attention to the sensations. Do not get caught up in the content of your thoughts but rather observe them as blips on a movie screen.

8. Next, move the focus of your attention as well as your hands to the rest of your upper body, including your breasts. Describe the sensations to yourself as you touch these parts of your body. Try on a positive sexual identity as you notice signs of vitality in these parts of your body. For the next few minutes, allow your attention to move fluidly to all of the different things that you are feeling in your body while maintaining the image of yourself, in your mind's eye, as a sexual and sensual woman. Do not worry if this image seems hard to believe in this moment.

9. Continue to do this for a few more minutes. Then gradually make the intention to move your hands and feet and slowly open your eyes. Take a moment to pay attention to how you feel as the exercise comes to an end.

If you notice negative thoughts arise at any point during this exercise, just take note of them ("Ah, judgmental thoughts are here"), and when they have faded away, redirect your attention back to your bodily sensations. Do not be hard on yourself if you find this difficult. Many women do, and it often takes some practice to feel comfortable with this exercise. We recommend that you try this exercise twice in the first week.

After subsequent practices, some women like to pair this exercise with a sexual aid such as fantasy, a vibrator, or erotica beforehand to first elicit a mild sexual arousal response. You may notice that if you first elicit some sexual arousal, adopting a positive sexual image comes a little bit more easily, and then your ability to notice sensations in your body, including your genitals, also comes about a little more easily.

Whether you have experienced a clinical depression or not, you will most likely face sadness or the blues at some point in your life. And you may be like the countless women for whom a sad mood dampens sexual desire. Mindfulness is an invaluable skill for identifying the beginning of a downward trajectory in mood and for helping you to manage more significant symptoms of depression when they surface. Mindfulness also offers a way to remain in the present moment and to keep from living in the past. There is a certain safety in being with whatever you are feeling right now. It is about welcoming all of the guests at the door, because each one has been sent as a guide from beyond.

CHAPTER 8

IT TAKES TWO

"Whatever kind of sex works for two (or more) individuals will be more enticing if the partners are alive, embodied and integrated within themselves and absorbed in and engaged with one another in the moment."

PEGGY KLEINPLATZ, in *Treating Sexual Desire Disorders: A Clinical Casebook*

S HARON ARRIVED HOME early from work so that she could prepare dinner and have the kids fed and put to bed early. It was a Friday night—the night that she and her husband, James, had set aside as a date night every week, when they could be alone, without their three children. The scheduled time was not necessarily for sexual activity but was intended to protect time so that they could have a bath together or an intimate massage. Nevertheless, Sharon and James had engaged in sexual activity on their previous two date nights, and she anticipated that the same might happen again this week.

Sharon had been struggling with her level of motivation for sex over the past five years, but it was only in the past ten months that she had decided it was time for her and her husband to address this sticking point in their otherwise (mostly) happy relationship. In working with a counselor, they had explored Sharon's tendency to feel overwhelmed when James's voice was slightly louder than usual. Sharon worked on being more assertive in expressing her needs while James worked on cultivating empathy for Sharon's experiences, identifying triggers for his own anger, and using less destructive ways of behaving than yelling when his anger took hold of him. They responded well to counseling, and both made concrete changes in their behavior that were recognized and praised by the other partner. Their relationship seemed to be on an upswing.

On this particular Friday night, after the children were asleep, Sharon put fresh sheets on her bed and slipped on a new silk nightie she had bought. She felt anxious but reminded herself of her commitment to working on her relationship with James; protecting these Friday night dates was important for fulfilling this commitment. James entered the room and appeared preoccupied. He began to talk about a confrontation with a colleague at work, speaking in a belittling manner about his coworker. As he spoke, Sharon's anxiety mounted. She could not empathize with James and instead imagined being in the shoes of James's coworker, who, Sharon believed, was the recipient of unwarranted and aggressive name-calling by James. Although James focused his comments on the interaction with his coworker, Sharon could imagine James directing these criticisms at her. She remembered a time a few years ago when he had humiliated her at a Christmas party in front of her friends by continuing to tell an embarrassing story despite noticing tears welling up in her eyes. In that moment of listening to James rant about this work situation, she felt overwhelmed with feelings of sadness, anxiety, and resentment.

She walked out of the room, whispering as she left, "I need to go now."

Unfortunately, an unpleasant exchange with a partner can derail a date night—even one that had been intricately planned and pleasantly anticipated, as was the situation with Sharon and James. A relationship provides a rich font of emotions for partners—the love and pride that partners experience in a relationship is unrivaled in other relationships, but at the other end of the spectrum, emotional conflict can be a source of extreme distress in couples and is often the focus of couples therapy. Some psychological therapies for couples, such as emotion-focused therapy, emphasize the importance of identifying and expressing emotions. The creators of emotion-focused therapy describe it as a way to help couples "accept, express, regulate, make sense of, and transform emotion." As emotions surface in a therapy session, couples are encouraged to identify and observe them and to try to understand what beliefs underlie a particular emotion. For example, a feeling of frustration may be related to an underlying belief such as "My partner does not listen to me—ever!" Labeling emotions and identifying the beliefs that are related to those emotions and that arise within a conflict can be extremely useful, since you may feel an emotion but not understand where it came from, why it is so intense, or why you are feeling that particular emotion and not another one (for example, why do I feel frustration and not sadness?).

Unlike emotion-focused therapy, which seeks to change emotions once they have been identified, mindfulness, as has been discussed throughout this book, is about bringing awareness and acceptance of whatever arises, including emotions. It is not about changing emotions—even if they are intensely unpleasant and unwanted. Often we engage in a

Ping-Pong match of hurtful statements with a partner, with each subsequent statement chipping away a little more at the emotional well-being of the other person. When that happens we are more likely to make comments that we would usually hold back when we are feeling less heated. In such situations, regret often quickly follows. An initial feeling of confusion can easily slip into feelings of hurt, then disappointment, discouragement, and hopelessness. And often this scenario unfolds within a few seconds. Multiply this by two, with each partner experiencing their own spiral of emotions, and you end up with a situation where emotional overload makes respectful communicating nearly impossible.

Relationship expert and researcher Dr. John Gottman describes this situation as diffuse physiological arousal, which impairs the functioning of the part of the brain responsible for empathy, problem solving, and overall conflict management. Gottman encourages couples to take some time for the emotions to ease off, on average about twenty minutes, before re-engaging in the conversation. In other words, when emotions become acutely and intensely activated to this point, further communication becomes ineffective and, in fact, may worsen the situation between partners. It's not difficult to imagine that bringing attention back to the present moment, instead of being side-tracked in defensive moves, might be especially useful for helping couples to respectfully resolve a conflict.

MINDFULNESS FOR COUPLES

THERE ARE APPROACHES to mindfulness that have been specifically adapted for couples to improve their relationship. If one partner is taught to be more mindful of their own internal processes, they become more aware of the presence of their partner, which in turn increases the likelihood that they will understand their partner's point of view. This may then lead them to respond in less judgmental and reactive ways. By becoming more mindful and more aware of the emotional impact of a conflict on themselves and their partner, they can learn to respond more positively to one another. It turns out that mindfulness allows us to be aware of both emotions and also the sometimes knee-jerk reactions we exhibit toward a partner when we feel particular strong emotions. And just as we have been using mindfulness skills to become aware of the breath and body, we can use those same skills to become aware of how we feel.

There is an entire field of science devoted to studying emotional intelligence, which refers to an ability not only to manage your own emotions but also to understand and influence the emotions of others. Research into emotional intelligence shows that when we see a change in a partner's facial expression or behavior, it takes only $\frac{1}{200}$ second for us to register that emotion. In such cases, it can be tempting to react automatically to what the other person said or did. However, by practicing mindfulness on our own, and by becoming experienced in noting our own feelings and thoughts in the present moment without judgment, we may become better at adjusting our reactions to a partner before our own emotions become so acutely and intensely activated that we are unable to communicate respectfully.

What does this actually look like? A couple can practice mindfulness together, sitting or lying side by side, for example, using the Body Scan. We can take note of when the mind wanders away from the body and toward thoughts or judgments with a partner just as we do while practicing on our own. With a partner present, though, we may be more prone to slipping into thoughts such as, "What is my partner thinking? Are they finding this boring?" If this happens, we can redirect attention back onto the bodily sensations and let negative thoughts "just be."

Another option was offered by psychologists Agnes Kocsis and John Newbury-Helps at St. Mary's Hospital in London. They developed a six-week program called Mindfulness in Sex Therapy and Intimate Relationships in which group members do a mindful exercise in pairs. In an exercise called back-to-back sensing, partners sit or stand back to back and bring the same qualities of mindful attention and nonjudgment to noticing their partner's body. Here is the exercise, in case you and your partner would like to try it.

Back-to-Back Sensing

Sit (or stand if that is more comfortable) on the ground, back to back with your partner. There will be points of contact between your bodies. For about fifteen minutes, notice what sensations arise in your own body. Notice the points of contact between your two bodies. Try to move your awareness even closer into those sensations. If you feel a need to move because you are uncomfortable, try to move intentionally and with an attitude of caring about and for the other person. After the fifteen minutes, move so that you are facing one another and answer the following questions:

- Was there any feeling of intimacy in relation to feeling your partner's body?
- How was being aware of your partner's body related to your own awareness of emotions and thoughts?

- Did you notice any sounds during this exercise, either yours or those of your partner?
- How did becoming aware of sounds impact the experience for you?

Another practice common in mindfulness-based relationship enhancement programs is loving kindness meditation—also known as Metta in the Pali language. In loving kindness meditation, the practice begins with noticing a love for oneself by following this instruction: "Begin by generating this kind feeling toward yourself. Notice any areas of self-judgment, then say, 'May I be free from harm. May I be safe and protected. May I be happy. May I be healthy and strong.'" After cultivating a love for oneself, one invites a pure and unconditional love for a partner: "May my partner be safe and unharmed. May they feel love. May they be safe, happy, healthy, and live joyously." In this program, one option is to practice yoga with a partner, with partners physically supporting one another during each pose, while each one pays attention to what it feels like to touch and to be touched.

In a 2004 study from the University of North Carolina at Chapel Hill, an eight-session mindfulness-based program to improve relationships was found to lead to significant improvements in couples' happiness, the amount of stress in their relationship, their ability to overcome stress when it arises, and overall stress. Mindfulness not only changed a partner's behavior during conflict but also enhanced their ability to understand the other person's behavior and respond in a manner that conveyed equanimity, or composure and evenness, during times of conflict. In addition, on the day that partners practiced mindfulness, and for the next few days afterward, they experienced significantly greater happiness in their relationship, highlighting the tangible day-to-day effects of mindfulness. Improvements were related to the amount of practice the couples did during the eight-week program, with most couples averaging about thirty minutes of mindful practice at home daily.

MINDFULNESS AND CORTISOL, THE STRESS HORMONE

ONE OF THE ways in which mindfulness may affect a couple's behavior is through its influence on the primary stress hormone, cortisol. In a study from the University of Oregon in 2016, couples were brought into a lab, given a topic of conflict, and asked to have a conversation about it. They provided saliva samples of cortisol before and after their conversation. The researchers found that practicing mindfulness during the conflict led to better cortisol recovery afterward, meaning that the participants' cortisol returned more quickly to a pre-stress level. However, how quickly cortisol levels returned to normal also depended on the type of conflict being discussed and on the intensity of a partner's negative behavior. Whereas mindfulness allowed participants to remain more engaged during low-intensity conflict, more severe forms of conflict were more difficult for mindfulness to manage. This suggests that mindfulness, by itself, may not be enough to ameliorate the impact of highly destructive forms of conflict.

Returning to Sharon and James, if Sharon had been able to convey empathy toward James, it is possible that he may have, in turn, felt some empathy toward his colleague. Such a response can help moderate levels of cortisol during an intense argument.

Kocsis and Newbury-Helps suggest an exercise to directly target empathy, which they call mindful listening (described below). Listening mindfully can be especially important for those who expect their partners to read their minds. Have you ever been in a relationship with someone—perhaps your current partner—and found yourself thinking, "This person should know what I like without my having to tell them. After all, we have been together for so many years!" The mind-reading fallacy, which maintains that we often believe our partners should know our thoughts and preferences without our explicitly stating them, is a common feature in many North American bedrooms and leads people to not tell their partner what they really want. We believe our partners *should* know, and if they do not, we see it as a symptom of relationship conflict or doom. It seems that our continuing faith in the mind-reading fallacy (that my partner *should* know, that the ability to mind-read my partner's preferences is an indicator of a better-adjusted relationship) is getting in the way of our experiencing true sexual pleasure. We also fear hurting our partners if we ask them to do something different from what they have been doing for years, sometimes decades. When we practice listening mindfully, we learn to better appreciate both the verbal and nonverbal messages from our partner, instead of making assumptions about what they are thinking or feeling. It may also be that mindfulness contributes to such conversations between a couple being less stressful, with perhaps less cortisol secreted by each partner.

Mindful Listening

This exercise guides you to notice how you are in this moment. You and your partner will take turns talking and listening. Start by deciding who is going to speak first (Person 1) and who is going to listen (Person 2).

1. Person 1 will share their experience of what they are noticing. Person 2 listens without talking but will also notice what sensations emerge in their own body and what thoughts arise. Person 2 may notice their reactions to Person 1 as well. Both of you should try to notice what comes up moment by moment. As you encounter periods of silence, notice that too. Don't move into a conversation at that point but instead sit with the silence until something arises for Person 1 to share.

2. After two to five minutes, Person 2 will share what it was like to listen mindfully. They may also ask any questions they wish about Person 1's experience. This is an opportunity to show curiosity about Person 1's experience, but it is not a conversation. Silence may occur, and if so, just notice it. This should continue for about two minutes.

3. Next, Persons 1 and 2 will reverse roles, and Person 2 will now share their experience of what they notice for about two to five minutes. They may share what sensations they notice in their body or in their mind. Person 1 will listen mindfully and notice what arises for them as they listen without interrupting. At the end of this period, Person 1 will have the opportunity to discuss what it was like to listen mindfully and to ask any questions of Person 2, drawn from their own curiosity. This will continue for two minutes.

At the end of the formal exercise, you may debrief with one another and consider the following questions:

- Did you notice any experience of connection?
- What was it like to listen and communicate mindfully?
- What was your sense of self in relation to your partner?
- Did you notice any kindness when you were just listening?
- Were you aware of any needs you had?
- Did you experience any discomfort?

THE ROLE OF FEELINGS

HOW MIGHT THESE exercises in noticing a partner's body, listening mindfully, and showing curiosity about a partner's experience be relevant to a couple's sexuality? Because sex is typically interactive, exercises designed to make one person aware of the impact of their own behavior or words on the other person's behavior, words, and feelings are entirely relevant. The dynamics of a relationship, including how the woman feels about her partner, how much she likes or admires her partner, and what she believes about the likely fate of their relationship, are major predictors of that woman's sexual desire.

In the large British NATSAL study carried out between 2010 and 2012, people experiencing sexual difficulties were 2.4 times as likely to not find it easy to talk to a partner about sex, and 2.9 times as likely to be unhappy in their relationship. In a 2008 study from the University of Melbourne, Australia, that measured women's sex-related distress, feelings for a partner, mood, and other psychosocial variables longitudinally over eleven years, the researchers found that feeling distress because of sex was strongly affected by a woman's negative feelings toward her partner. Moreover, a woman's negative feelings for her partner over many years were identified as the most significant predictor of her level of sex-related distress many years later. This also means that a woman's feelings toward her partner can affect her sexual distress even a decade later.

It seems that a woman's feelings for her partner contribute more than anything else to her level of sexual desire. This relationship is bidirectional: low sexual desire reduces a woman's satisfaction with her relationship as well as her partner's level of satisfaction with their relationship and their sexual life.

INTEGRATING MINDFULNESS INTO
YOUR SEXUAL RELATIONSHIP

IN OUR MINDFULNESS group program at the University of British Columbia, women begin by practicing mindfulness on their own for at least a month in a nonsexual situation and without a partner. As discussed earlier, we spend much of the time in our face-to-face sessions practicing mindfulness, and then the women are provided with audiorecordings to continue their mindfulness practice at home between sessions.

By the time we shift to a discussion about how to incorporate mindfulness into their relationship with their partner, the women in our groups have established a solid mindfulness practice on their own. They have learned how to observe the activities of the mind and how to distance themselves from thoughts by labeling them "mental events." They begin to calmly resist the tendency to judge themselves for becoming distracted and instead view this distraction as a moment of mindfulness—when they catch themselves wrapped up in a cascade of thoughts, they give themselves a mental pat on the back and return their focus to the sensations arising in their body.

When we introduce mindfulness to a couple, we suggest that the women incorporate their skills in nonjudgmental awareness in the present moment directly into their sexual activities. As her partner touches her arms, her legs, and her back, we invite each woman to tune in to all of the individual sensations that emerge moment by moment. When she does this, she automatically slows down to notice the emerging sensations, such as the early twinges of arousal. She is encouraged to give those sensations a name and to adopt a stance of nonjudgmental acceptance, meaning that as she notices sensations in her body arising from contact with her partner, she can try to let go of judging those sensations as being "not strong enough," "not the same as last time," or "not satisfying to my partner."

Because this can be challenging, we encourage the women to become aware of their body as a whole, noticing, for example, its position, posture, and location. We also guide the women to use each of their five senses to observe whatever sensation is most prominent for them in that moment of being sexual. The following questions might be used to guide your focus of attention as you are engaging in sexual activity with a partner:

- What patterns of color, shape, or movement do you see as you look at your partner?
- At the points of contact between you and your partner, what temperature/pressure/texture/sensation do you experience?
- Do you notice sensations of movement, such as expansion/stretching/contraction in those parts of your body where you are making voluntary movements?
- What are the individual sounds that you hear as you breathe? Listen to your partner and notice any sounds. What do you hear when you vocalize?

We encourage the women to observe their sensations non-judgmentally and then to consider making adjustments to their posture, position, or actions if that is what feels right for them in the moment.

When the women learn to be right where they are when with a partner, rather than in the myriad other places that their mind escapes to during sex, they start to experience sexual contact with their partner in a way that perhaps they had not experienced for months, years, or decades. In fact, many women participating in our studies tell us that they feel like part of a dating couple again: one that is discovering touches and sensations for the first time.

In our studies of gynecologic cancer survivors who, at the beginning of our program, would tell us that they "feel nothing," we found that repeated practice of mindfulness skills, first alone and then during partnered sexual encounters, led them to notice sexual sensations that they had been missing (or perhaps ignoring?) because they were mourning the loss associated with the physical changes due to their cancer treatment. We did not attempt to invalidate their experiences of loss, particularly since many of these women experienced new physical challenges associated with a radical hysterectomy, radiation therapy, or a rapid decline in hormones due to chemotherapy. However, as we gently and repeatedly guided them back to their own moment-by-moment sensations, they gradually realized that they did not "feel nothing." Yes, the sexual sensations of some of the women felt different from their sensations before their cancer treatment, but they also experienced hope that by relating to their sensations in this new and more mindful way, they could become curious again—even excited again—about the ways in which their body responded to a partner's touch.

In Kocsis and Newbury-Helps's six-session Mindfulness in Sex Therapy and Intimate Relationships Program, group participants experienced first-hand the role of mindfulness in helping them address their own avoidance of sex by first becoming aware of their need for sex to be a certain way and then recognizing how having this sexual goal could provoke sex-related distress. Once they let go of their sexual goal and focused, instead, on moment-by-moment sensations, they could move their awareness onto the sensations themselves. The more one pays attention, the more the brain becomes activated—especially those centers that play a role in bodily awareness (like the insula), which may further boost sexual response. As we've seen in earlier chapters, mindfulness allows those emotional centers of the brain, which may elicit negative or judgmental feelings, to remain quiet.

A team of Australian sex researchers has adapted our and others' face-to-face mindfulness programs to an online format and administered it to couples in which the woman was experiencing significant sexual difficulties. The program, known as Pursuing Pleasure, consists of six online modules, each approximately two weeks apart. The mindfulness exercises are very brief (only five minutes each), and participants practice them every day. In addition to the online modules, participants have unlimited email access to the facilitator in case they have questions that are not covered in the program's online questions and answers section.

Those who took part in Pursuing Pleasure saw an increase in their sexual intimacy, emotional intimacy, and communication scores, which were also significantly greater than those of participants in a control group. Three months after completing the program, the couples had maintained their improvements in emotional intimacy and communication, but there was some deterioration in their levels of sexual intimacy. It is possible that six sessions is not enough for long-term changes in sexual intimacy or that the effects of an online program might have been boosted by some face-to-face contact with a facilitator. Because sexual intimacy can be affected by many factors, it may be that mindfulness alone is not sufficient to address other areas of conflict in a relationship that contribute to poor sexual intimacy. Nonetheless, this research offers hope to couples like Sharon and James, who may quickly spiral into emotionally charged conflict, that bringing awareness to the present moment may be an effective means of fostering both emotional and sexual intimacy, and a way of breaking the vicious cycle of communication blockade.

Sensate focus is another couple-focused mindfulness exercise that is potent for both cultivating awareness and helping partners to recognize the expectations and judgments that arise in the bedroom and that directly affect sexual response. In the earlier section about the sex therapy pioneers Masters and Johnson, we saw that they believed that sex was a natural function and that sensate focus formed the cornerstone of sex therapy. They also believed that as a natural function, sexual arousal (which includes lubrication, erections, and orgasm) was an involuntary process that could be influenced by voluntary factors but only after a lengthy period of training. In part, they believed that sexual arousal could not be influenced because it originated from lower, limbic areas of the brain that were not under our voluntary control.

Because they believed that many sexual difficulties arose from performance anxiety, they also believed that the key to an effective treatment was to mitigate those anxieties by redirecting a patient's attention to their sensory experience and helping them to focus on behaviors that were under their voluntary control. As detailed in Weiner and Avery-Clark's book *Sensate Focus in Sex Therapy: The Illustrated Manual*, Masters and Johnson observed three unique features of their research subjects who responded with sexual ease: (1) they touched a partner for their own experience, not for their partner's, (2) they focused on the sensations associated with touching rather than on a wish to arouse their partner, and (3) when distracted, they would continually redirect their attention back to the sensations of touch. They described this as nondemand touching. The goal is not to elicit pleasurable feelings but rather to observe any feelings that arise.

If you have not tried sensate focus already, now is an ideal time to do so with a partner. Whether you are in a new or long-term relationship, sensate focus may be a way to experience your partner's touch in an entirely new way.

Sensate Focus Exercise

Phase 1
Sensate focus is a structured, progressive exercise designed for couples that consists of three phases. In Phase 1, one partner touches the other partner from head to toes, excluding the genitals and breasts/chest, and the receiver of the touch focuses on their own sensations. By experiencing your own sensations and redirecting your attention continually back to those sensations if, for example, you start to worry about your partner's reactions, any expectations you have about becoming aroused are deactivated. Paradoxically, when you do this, you may become more likely to feel sexually aroused. But because we often default to "thinking" ("I hope my partner likes this" or "I hope I am doing this right"), we often need to

be encouraged over and over again to focus purely on sensations and to understand that the arousal will come later.

After about fifteen minutes, the roles are reversed: the person receiving the touch now does the touching, and the person giving the touch now becomes the receiver. Eventually, both of you may come to feel that you are able to redirect the focus of attention onto sensations, that the tendency to drift into a sea of negative judgments lessens, and that when negative thoughts arise, you are able to move in and quickly redirect attention back to the sensations that emerge during touch. Some couples are able to attain this after a few trials of sensate focus, and other couples may need much more practice.

Phase 2
After you have practiced Phase 1 a few times, you may feel ready to progress to Phase 2. In this phase, all areas of the body may be touched, including the genitals, the chest, and any other erogenous zones that were off-limits in Phase 1. Otherwise, the process is identical to that followed in Phase 1. As Weiner and Avery-Clark note in their book, you might choose to focus on temperature, texture, and pressure, because these are powerful portals into the longed-for sexual arousal and pleasure. However, eliciting sexual arousal, as in Phase 1, is still not the goal of the touching. The goal is to truly attain mindfulness.

Phase 3
There is a third phase to sensate focus that Masters and Johnson developed but that has not been described so far in this book. Instead of the one-person-at-a-time protocol that was followed in Phases 1 and 2, during Phase 3 there is mutual

touching in any location and in any position that the giver of the touch wishes. As one is giving and receiving touch at the same time, both partners may experiment with shifting the focus of their attention back and forth from the sensations of being touched to those of giving touch while noticing the vibrations of contact when they are being touched and the warmth of their fingertips as they touch their partner's chest, legs, and everywhere else on the body. By slowing down, they can move their attention from these different locations at their own pace. You may be interested in experimenting with this yourself.

In more advanced stages of Phase 3, one partner may lie on top of the other so that there is genital-to-genital contact. Given the richness of the touch receptors in the genitals, one can also focus on how the genitals feel to give touch and to receive touch. With time, one can also focus attention on sensations that arise as penetration occurs, noticing what penetration feels like without any thrusting movements for both the giver and the receiver. Both opposite-sex and same-sex couples may perform this exercise (in the case of a woman partnered with a woman, a strap-on dildo may facilitate penetration). By using the power of mindfulness, a once familiar practice (sex) can be transformed to become entirely new and exciting again.

Like mindfulness, sensate focus was not intended to elicit relaxation or positive feelings, but inevitably it did so. Although Masters and Johnson did not refer to sensate focus as a mindfulness practice, you can quickly glean from the instructions above that it is very much an application of mindfulness. Some of the instructions that Masters and Johnson gave to their clients include "Pay attention to the sensations as your partner touches your body," "Don't worry about the outcome," and "Focus on the tactile sensations such as temperature, pressure, and texture." They reasoned that focusing on one's own sensations and *not* on arousal or performance was a necessary step toward sexual pleasure and resolution of symptoms like anxiety. Focusing attention on sensations of the body, redirecting attention from distractions and worries back to the body, and not trying to create a certain *type* of experience for the receiver are all the same elements of mindfulness that we have been discussing. Perhaps it is because of sensate focus's ability to cultivate mindfulness—and the power mindfulness holds for experiencing the multitude of sensations in the present moment—that it remains one of the most frequently used tools in sex therapy.

In 2003, at the University of Washington, I codeveloped an intervention that would teach cancer survivors how to pay attention to their bodies and how to release the grip of cancer-related worries and judgments about their sexual difficulties, using the term "mindfulness" to describe the program. Many experts in the field saw this as a new addition to the armamentarium of therapeutic techniques available to sex therapists. But Masters and Johnson deserve credit for originally developing the theory that cultivating present-moment awareness, with a focus on the body, is so important to healthy sexual functioning. They truly were the original brains behind achieving better sex through mindfulness.

Could Sharon and James (and couples like them) bene- fit from mindfulness, and could they engage in this practice together? If so, Sharon might recognize that her disappointment in their planned date night had arisen from her belief that James should have known the immense effort she had put into it and that he should not have "killed the mood" by complaining about his coworker. Sharon might have noticed these thoughts and engaged with them as "events of the mind" rather than as an indication that James did not care about the great effort Sharon had put into planning the date night. She might then have asked James if he would consider putting the unpleasant work encounter on the shelf until the next day so that they could enjoy their time together. James, too, might have behaved differently had he observed when he arrived home that Sharon had been busy planning a quiet evening for them. Rather than re-enacting the unpleasant encounter over and over again in his mind, and then telling Sharon about it, James might have observed the look of anticipation in Sharon's eyes when he walked in the door.

Both Sharon and James were easily swept up in a cascade of thoughts, and for Sharon, this was particularly true during sexual activity. When James touched her during foreplay, she worried about becoming sexually aroused, as she did not want to disappoint him. Her focus during sex for years had been on keeping James satisfied, to the detriment of her own experience. By remaining focused on ensuring that the encounter was pleasurable for James, Sharon frequently bypassed kissing, touching, caressing, and foreplay in general, even though earlier in their relationship she had welcomed an hour of this type of physical intimacy. She used to love kissing, and in her own words, the world "seemed to stop" when she kissed James.

The combination of mindful listening, back-to-back sensing, and sensate focus exercises allowed Sharon and James to feel body sensations and emotions, without expectations and without the need to elicit a certain type of response that they believed their partner wanted. Becoming aware of her own sensations during the touch exchanges of sensate focus provided the conduit to her sexual pleasure that Sharon had been missing for years. Moreover, by restricting the exercise to nonerotic touch, and prohibiting sexual activity immediately afterward, Sharon felt motivated for sex for the first time in decades. Observing her bodily sensations gave rise to feelings of pleasure, which in turn gave her a renewed desire for sex. She also came to realize how important nonsexual touch and foreplay were for her, both because they slowed down the encounter and because they were very pleasing.

After approximately four months of practicing mindfulness together and incorporating sensate focus, the quality of their encounters, as rated by both Sharon and James, increased dramatically. James no longer took his work into every aspect of his home life, and he developed a deeper sense of empathy for Sharon. This allowed him to understand and validate Sharon for what she was experiencing in the moment instead of his previous tendency to launch into his own stories.

Mindfulness is a powerful tool for cultivating awareness and for experiencing events at their fullest. In the same way that we have been bringing mindful awareness to sensations in our bodies and minds with the Body Scan and the mindfulness of thoughts practice, we can bring that same attention to sensations experienced during contact with a partner. My hope is that the exercises in this chapter will help you feel alive sexually again and, if you are in a relationship, that this aliveness permeates all points of contact between you and your partner.

CHAPTER 9

TUNING IN TO PAIN

Pain is inevitable. Suffering is optional.

BUDDHIST PROVERB

ALTHOUGH LOW SEXUAL desire is the most common sex-related concern for women, for approximately 15 percent of North American women, excruciatingly painful sex is a regular occurrence. This is not the discomfort that often occurs the first time a woman experiences vaginal penetration or the tenderness that may accompany hormonal changes as a result of breastfeeding or menopause, but a sharp, shooting, and cutting pain that occurs with even the slightest amount of contact with the vagina. And it is evident why sex that is painful would ultimately extinguish your interest in sex.

Sierra is a twenty-six-year-old woman who has been in a committed, monogamous relationship for the past three years. Although Sierra had numerous boyfriends throughout high school and college, she ended these relationships when her partners started to nudge the relationship toward increasing sexual activity. She thoroughly enjoyed mutual oral sex,

kissing, and petting, but she had never engaged in sexual intercourse. Before she met Ali, her partners would withdraw from
the relationship when Sierra insisted that sexual intercourse
would not happen until marriage. Ali was different. She met
him at the college library when she was twenty-three years old,
and they quickly bonded over the fact that they were midway
through their master's degrees in biology. They had an intense
affection for one another, as well as deep respect for one another's career ambitions. They fell in love within a few months,
and Sierra would enjoy spending hours kissing and caressing
Ali. In the first few months of their relationship, they never
spoke about sexual intercourse, but Sierra alluded to "gynecologic concerns" she had experienced since she was a teenager
and mentioned that she had never had a Pap smear or a genital
examination by a physician. After about four months of dating,
Ali and Sierra felt certain about their love for one another, and
they agreed to consummate their relationship while they were
visiting a remote and idyllic coastal island.

Sierra anticipated the evening for several weeks, imagining
the night's events in detail. On the planned evening, the couple had a beautiful night that included a long walk, a delicious
dinner, and wine. They kissed on the boardwalk overlooking
the Pacific Ocean and held hands as they watched the sun set.
Everything was perfect. They returned to their luxurious hotel
room and kissed, as they usually did, for hours.

The moment came when Ali was ready to penetrate Sierra.
"Are you ready?" he asked. To which she replied, "I think so.
But please go ahead slowly." At the moment Ali's penis met
Sierra's vulva, she experienced an extreme anxiety reaction,
feeling as if her "vagina was closing up," and she pushed him
away. Understandably, this puzzled both of them, particularly
since everything that evening had seemed perfect. Her anxiety

made no sense to her. How could she love someone so much and have such a strong phobic reaction to his coming close to her? Ali's reaction was warm, empathic, and understanding. "It's OK," he said. "We don't have to do this if you're not ready." Instead, they fell asleep in one another's arms. The next night they tried again. And Sierra had a similar response: anxiety, fear, and emotional distress.

PVD: WHEN SEX HURTS

TWO WEEKS LATER, Sierra's family doctor confirmed the diagnosis: provoked vestibulodynia (PVD). PVD leads a woman to experience extreme pain when the vulvar vestibule (the area of a woman's genitals which includes the vulva and vagina) is touched in any way. The diagnosis of PVD is made when other reasons for the genital pain are ruled out: conditions such as vulvar-vaginal atrophy related to menopause, skin conditions such as lichen sclerosis, or vulvar dysplasias or cancer. A physician uses a cotton swab to lightly touch different areas around the vulva and vagina and the patient self-reports which locations elicit a very high level of pain, compared with areas around the thigh or labia majora, which are not painful or sensitive. Although considerable research focused on the nature and causes of PVD has been published, there is still so much more we do not know, and this leaves care providers in a conundrum about the best way of managing this distressing pain and caring for women who suffer from it.

Like Sierra, many women with PVD attribute their vaginal pain to inexperience. "Maybe it is supposed to hurt the first few times?" they ask themselves and their friends. But when the pain persists, regardless of how long they have been in a relationship, how much emotional closeness there is in the relationship, how aroused they feel, or how much "foreplay" has occurred before penetration is attempted, the women eventually realize that their pain is not normal. Trying to relax during sex appears to make little difference, and as a result, many women with PVD will bypass foreplay and other typically pleasurable activities in order to get to intercourse quickly and get it over with.

For years, PVD was understood to be a superficial pain caused by a vulvar skin sensitivity, a local infection or inflammation, or vaginal trauma. As a result, treatment entailed topical ointments. Although some women experienced some benefit from these treatments, including steroid creams lathered directly on the vulva and in the vagina, the majority of women with vulvar pain did not benefit, and a subset even experienced a worsening of symptoms, compounding not only their pain but also their distress associated with feeling broken and abnormal.

Many women who experience intense vaginal pain like Sierra's suffer in silence for years before receiving an accurate diagnosis. Sierra was fortunate to have a physician who readily recognized her intense fear of vaginal pain and the pain itself as PVD. However, other women may end up meeting with many different health-care providers, each of whom promises to improve the vulvar pain, but at best delivers minimal improvement.

Sierra's first experience with vaginal pain from sex was with Ali. However, for years before that she had experienced pain with vaginal contact from attempting to use a tampon, and she took it upon herself to completely eliminate all forms of irritants, including soap, aromatic laundry detergents, and anything but cotton underwear. She tracked the frequency and intensity of her pain as she continued to try to use tampons, and although some degree of pain with vaginal touch was present most of the time, she found that the intensity varied anywhere from a 10 out of 10 (imagine the worst pain you could ever endure) to a 1 out of 10 (a mild pain, more of an annoyance). She noticed that during times of stress and anxiety (especially around the time she was preparing to defend her master's thesis), her pain became so unbearable that, on some days, she could only lie on her couch with her legs spread to ensure that nothing came into contact with her vulva.

After Sierra discovered that her vaginal pain from tampons also extended to her attempts to have intercourse, and after continuing to try intercourse for some time, she experienced a sharp decline in her desire for sex. She avoided undressing in front of Ali so that she would not "turn him on" and then reject his invitation for sex. Her desire for nonintercourse forms of intimacy also plummeted, as did her desire for the hours of kissing and petting she used to enjoy. Nine months into the relationship, Sierra tried to break up with Ali, insisting that he did not deserve to be with someone who could not enjoy sexual intercourse with pleasure and without pain.

For many years, treatment of women like Sierra was entirely medical—using either topical creams or oral medications in the belief that the vulvar pain was due to an injury or trauma to the area and that the ongoing pain was a result of an increased sensitization of pain nerve endings in the area. This supposition is partially true—for many women with PVD, an initial triggering event can set off a cascade of events that leave the woman in chronic genital pain, and biopsies of women with PVD show a high level of innervation of pain nerve endings in that area. But this view is incomplete, and it led researchers to explore what else could be contributing to this vulvar pain when there was no evidence that the cause of the pain was due to a physical trauma.

Major advances in the understanding and treatment of women with PVD only occurred after researchers started to focus their efforts on the brain. There is now evidence that PVD acts like other chronic pain conditions in that its symptoms are perpetuated because of changes in the brain's pain system. Imagine a house alarm that is triggered when the wind blows as opposed to when an intruder breaks in. This analogy is helpful for understanding how a woman experiences vulvar pain when only a slight touch (or sometimes even no touch at all) is applied to the vulva—a stimulus that most women would not perceive as painful, and some may not even notice at all. But the brain of a woman with PVD registers the light touch as a painful stimulus, eliciting a cascade of neuronal events as if the woman had come into contact with a painful stimulus. In other words, the brain reacts to the light touch as if it were a sharp object.

But what causes the brain to do this in the first place? The phenomenon known as central sensitization explains what happens to the neurons in the brain to allow nonpainful stimuli to be experienced as painful. Central sensitization means that the brain and spinal cord get "wound up" and are in a persistent state of reactivity, which lowers the threshold for detecting pain. The exact reasons underlying why some people develop central sensitization and others do not are not entirely clear. However, it is known that genetics may play a role. There is also evidence that psychological factors—such as how readily one launches a stress response, anxiety levels, and a history of depression—can make someone more vulnerable to developing central sensitization and chronic pain.

Medical treatments like topical creams and oral medications are commonly prescribed by gynecologists to help women alleviate their vulvar pain. But purely medical treatments have not been able to adequately address the degree of suffering experienced by women like Sierra. Feelings of sexual incompetence and lack of desirability, guilt about an unsatisfying sex life for a partner, fears that her situation will never improve and that she will be alone forever, and feelings of hopelessness and helplessness are all layered on top of the woman's pain. Although women in relationships suffer, in part because of guilt that they are "depriving" their partners of a happy sex life, women who are not in a relationship face unique challenges: How can I tell someone that I can't have sex because it hurts? Who would want to be with someone who hates sex? Unfortunately, the most commonly prescribed treatments do not alleviate the enormous burden of suffering that women with PVD experience and, in some cases, may even make the symptoms—both the physical and the emotional ones—worse because the women do not experience satisfactory improvements in pain intensity.

Like other people who experience chronic pain, women with PVD have much higher rates of anxiety and depression than people without chronic pain. Furthermore, their tendency to catastrophize ("This is the worst pain ever and I'll never be able to cope!") has been found in research studies to be related to the intensity of their pain and the amount of activation in the brain. Even anticipating the pain before any form of touch may be enough to elicit some of the brain changes associated with actually experiencing the pain itself. Put another way, expecting pain may trigger feelings of actual pain, even if the vulva has not come into contact with anything. The tendency to catastrophize, along with a history of anxiety and depression, makes women vulnerable to developing not only PVD but also other chronic pain conditions, such as chronic migraines or chronic low back pain, and catastrophizing over symptoms is characteristic of most women who suffer from PVD.

Anyone imagining this situation for themselves can likely empathize with how stressful it must be. Dr. Rosemary Basson, who has been mentioned throughout this book for her thoughtful depiction of women's sexual response cycles, has also written extensively about the management of PVD. Basson argues that the stress associated with experiencing chronic vaginal pain itself contributes to the vicious cycle of pain. Drawing on a large body of science from the literature on other types of chronic pain, Basson maintains that the unique stress experienced by women with PVD leads directly to ongoing pain hypersensitivity in the brain. In addition to the factors that originally contributed to a woman's onset of genital pain, her experience of distress and suffering after weeks, months, and in many cases years, worsens the pain, and this can be traced back to changes in the brain's pain center. But Basson also argues that there is good news. Changes in the brain's pain circuits, and ultimately in a woman's experience of pain and associated sexual dysfunction, can be reversed. Furthermore, interrupting this vicious pain–sexual dysfunction–stress cycle may not even require medications or a visit to a gynecologist.

MINDFULNESS AS A TREATMENT FOR PVD

AT FIRST GLANCE, using mindfulness, with its emphasis on acceptance and compassion, seems counterintuitive for the treatment of genital pain. How could focusing on the pain lead to feeling better? After all, the pain is unwanted and distressing, and women may react negatively to the notion that they need to "just accept it." A deeper understanding of how mindfulness is applied to manage the pain of PVD is necessary in order to resolve this apparent paradox.

As discussed in Chapter 3, Jon Kabat-Zinn's first participants in his mindfulness-based stress reduction (MBSR) groups were people suffering from chronic and debilitating pain that had not responded to conventional treatments. After eight weeks of attending group mindfulness sessions and practicing mindfulness exercises such as the Body Scan at home between sessions, participants' sense of well-being, mood, quality of life, and even pain had improved. When those suffering from chronic pain learn mindfulness, they learn to cultivate a "decentered" approach to their thoughts; when thoughts arise, they practice viewing them simply as passing events of the mind rather than as facts, truths, or rules to be followed. When Buddhist monks' brains are scanned, the scans reveal evidence of less evaluation and emotional reactivity and a greater amount of attention paid to bare sensations than among nonmeditators. Brain imaging studies show that when meditators come into contact with a painful stimulus, their brains process it differently from the brains of nonmeditators, even if they are not meditating at the time. In other words, the benefits of mindfulness for chronic pain appear to persist even when meditators are not on the cushion.

Although mindfulness-based interventions have been used with people suffering from chronic pain for over forty years, they have only recently been applied to women experiencing chronic genital pain. Our team of researchers, sexual medicine physicians, and mindfulness experts at the University of British Columbia has developed, administered, and tested a mindfulness-based program for women suffering from chronic genital pain. Women in this program learn the same mindfulness exercises as the women seeking treatment for a sexual dysfunction. They learn to eat mindfully and to mindfully notice sensations while they are breathing, and they cultivate an awareness of sensations in their body.

The facilitators guide women with PVD to pay attention to their pain—the actual "bare sensations" that they experience during pain. Since women with PVD tend to experience their genital pain only when something comes into contact with their vulva or vagina, we do not ask them to elicit vulvar pain during their group sessions with us. Instead, we elicit pain during the session by asking the women to hold one hand straight up in the air. While holding a hand up might not sound like it would be painful, after about one minute this position starts to trigger a dull muscle soreness. At two minutes, this soreness becomes sharper and stings. And at the three-minute mark, the otherwise featherweight hand feels like a ton of bricks and the sharp pain starts to radiate down the shoulder blade and into the back and the rest of the body. Women who have existing pains elsewhere in their body (and that applies to most of us at some point) can focus on that area of discomfort for the duration of the in-session exercise.

In group, Sierra would be guided with questions: What are the qualities of the sensation? Where exactly do you experience them? Do the sensations come and go or wax and wane? Is there an emotional tone to the sensations when you experience them? Do the sensations extend to other areas? As you tune in to those bare sensations associated with pain, can you observe whether you have a tendency to want to ignore or move away from those sensations? And what happens to this aversion when you pay attention to it? And what about thoughts? When you have thoughts about the pain, can you view these thoughts as mental events? As something the mind does, as opposed to truths to be listened to?

For homework, the women are invited to provoke vulvar pain with their own fingers and practice the same mindful awareness of the bare sensations that they did when eliciting pain in their arm during the group sessions. If you experience vaginal or vulvar pain yourself, you might consider trying the following exercise at home. The object is not to see if the vulvar or vaginal pain has disappeared but rather to discover what happens when you are curious about and attentive to the sensations that make up the pain itself.

Provoking a Mild Genital Pain

In this exercise, you are first going to bring awareness to your body and to your breath before eliciting genital sensations. Some women may find provoking genital sensations too unpleasant. If so, feel free to use this practice as an opportunity to notice the sensations of your breath and your body without eliciting vulvar pain. You can also elicit pain elsewhere on your body or tune in to another area of pain that is already there.

1. Lie down in a comfortable position with your head propped up, ideally on a bed and in private. Take a moment to notice the points of contact between your body and the bed, and just notice what sensations you experience at those points of contact.

2. Bring your full attention to the sensations of breathing, noticing the in-breath and out-breath. Also notice where those sensations are experienced in your body. Perhaps

at your nostrils or your chest? Continue to practice awareness of your breath for about five to ten minutes.

3. Sooner or later, you'll notice that your mind has wandered
   off somewhere. This is not your fault, and it does not mean
   you are doing the exercise incorrectly. Just notice that it
   has occurred, and gently bring your attention back to your
   breath, putting it at the center of the field of your awareness. There is as much mindfulness in noticing that your
   mind has wandered off somewhere away from the breath
   as there is in continually paying attention to the sensations
   of breathing.

4. Moving slightly so that one hand will be able to move
   toward your genitals, see if you can focus on just one
   in-breath as you move your finger toward the vaginal
   opening. Can you just stay with one in-breath as you touch
   the area of the discomfort on the vulva? Stay in touch
   with your awareness for just that one in-breath. If you can
   do so, extend your awareness to the present sensations
   during an out-breath.

5. Touching the vagina, notice the intense physical sensations and let them just be on the periphery of your
   awareness, one breath at a time. As you continue to touch,
   the intense vulvar sensations may still be there, but focus
   your awareness on your breath. You're not trying to distract yourself from the discomfort or ignore the intense
   sensations. Rather, they are there on the periphery as you
   focus on being fully present as you observe the breath
   sensations; pain in the background, breath in the fore-
   ground. Continue to do this for the next five to ten minutes.

6. Next, you are going to move the focus of attention directly
   onto the painful sensations themselves. See if you can
   breathe into the region of the vulvar sensations, as if you

were directing your breath directly there. Moment by moment, as best as you can, allow the breath to bathe that region on each in-breath and then move away from it on the out-breath. Bring your full awareness to the sensations in that area as you touch it with your finger. As best you can, and with the lightest of touches, just observe what happens and see, in your mind's eye, what unfolds. Allow your breath to flow to the area of discomfort on each in-breath and to flow away from that area on each out-breath.

7. Could you experiment with not calling those sensations pain? This may feel strange, as we are accustomed to labeling something painful as "pain." But what if you could call it "intense physical sensations" instead? Try it now. What do you experience when you label the reaction as "pain"? And now what do you experience what you label the sensations as "intense physical sensations"? See if you can continue to label the sensations in this area as "intense physical sensations," not "pain," for about five to ten minutes.

You've just practiced noticing sensations of pain as part of a mindfulness practice. Peeking at the pain for just a second or two is still considered a form of tuning in to the pain and not avoiding it. Over time, you'll notice that your relationship with pain will change. For many women, the pain sensations themselves change and become less intense.

Scientific studies have demonstrated that it is much more effective to tune in to the sensations of pain themselves than to wall them off. Critical to this process is the "uncoupling" of the emotional, cognitive, and physiological components of pain, and there is evidence that as you learn to focus on the physiological components of pain (the bare sensations, as described in the practice you just did), the tendency to experience the pain symptoms as distressing lessens. Ultimately, as the proclivity to have a strong negative emotional and cognitive response to pain is reduced, it becomes experienced as less stressful. Brain scientists speculate that there is also less processing of the pain in the brain. The vicious cycle of pain and stress eventually dulls and perhaps is even interrupted. In a paradoxical way, tuning in to the pain leads to a tuning out of the distress it causes.

MUSCLES MATTER: PELVIC FLOOR PHYSIOTHERAPY AND MINDFULNESS

PELVIC FLOOR PHYSIOTHERAPY is another effective treatment for vulvar pain. This treatment is based on the finding that most women with PVD experience varying degrees of tension in their pelvic floor muscles as a result of their chronic genital or pelvic pain. The pelvic floor is the bed of muscles that provide support to the pelvic organs and prevent incontinence (leaking out of urine or feces). A healthy pelvic floor is necessary for proper bowel and bladder function but it can be damaged by a variety of factors, including pregnancy and delivery, aging, urogynecologic surgery, and pelvic organ prolapse. Among women with genital pain, there may be increased tone (tightness) in the pelvic floor muscles as well as a lack of control over when those muscles tighten involuntarily.

Pelvic floor physiotherapy is not typically delivered by a sports medicine physiotherapist but by physiotherapists who have undergone specialized training in the pelvic floor muscles. They spend most of their clinical time with patients accessing the pelvic floor. (Yes, access is provided by one of two orifices. You can guess which ones!) They use a variety of strategies to help women manage their vulvar pain, including education about pelvic floor control, biofeedback (which involves monitoring electrical signals that correspond to the amount of tension in the pelvic floor), and vaginal inserts of progressively increasing size, which are paired with relaxation, pelvic floor strengthening exercises, and a variety of manual techniques, including massage and stretching. Pelvic floor physiotherapy can be very effective for women with chronic vulvar or pelvic pain, though studies comparing its effects in the long term with those of psychological treatment find the latter results in better retention of gains.

Some experts advocate combining pelvic floor physiotherapy with mindfulness, since women can use mindfulness to confront negative thoughts that arise as they work through the various pelvic floor exercises. As the woman attempts to insert the smallest vaginal insert, she can practice mindfulness by first noticing all her physical sensations as the insert comes into contact with her body and then noticing any intense sensations or discomfort as she penetrates her vagina with the insert. She can also observe any thoughts that arise while paying attention to them as well as the myriad breath and body sensations. For example, when thoughts such as "This is so embarrassing to have to insert these objects into my vagina" occur, she can think, "There goes another judgment thought. Let me try to be kinder to myself and just notice whatever physical sensations arise." Or, as we practiced in the previous exercise, she can try to focus on the pain itself for just one breath and then move her attention elsewhere in the body.

DOES TUNING IN REDUCE GENITAL PAIN?

SO DOES MINDFULNESS work for women with genital or vulvar pain? One study found that compared with women who were assigned to a wait-list control condition during which they did not receive any treatment, women who underwent four sessions of group mindfulness-based therapy had significant reductions in genital pain, an improved sense of control over their pain, and far fewer psychological symptoms such as catastrophizing, hypervigilance (that is, being overly attuned to any changes in pain intensity), sex-related distress, and depression. These effects were still detected when the women were tested six months later. Feedback from the participants revealed that they no longer felt isolated and they had far more hope about their intimate relationships. Some women even commented that PVD had allowed them to consider other means of being sexual and that they had once again learned to feel arousal and to crave sexual activity that was not painful.

TUNING IN OR TURNING OFF THOUGHTS?

ON THE BASIS of these promising findings, our team carried out a five-year study in which we compared the effectiveness of eight sessions of group mindfulness with that of eight sessions of group cognitive behavioral therapy (CBT) for women with PVD. Several studies have found CBT to be effective for helping reduce genital pain and improving quality of life, and it has become a standard component of care globally for women with PVD. Many hospital-based programs are based on a multidisciplinary model in which teaching women skills in CBT is a core aspect.

As discussed in Chapter 2, CBT involves teaching the women skills so that they can identify "irrational" thoughts, such as "My partner will leave me if we don't have sex." Once the irrational thought is identified, the woman weighs the evidence to support the thought with the evidence that counters the thought to decide whether it is rational or irrational. When the evidence favors a more rational thought ("Even though I *feel* like my partner will leave me because of the pain, I know this is not true and they have reassured me that they are committed to me"), the woman is encouraged to try to replace the original catastrophic thought with this more rational one. With mindfulness, there is no attempt to challenge or change thoughts.

Which is better: CBT strategies aimed at challenging and changing thoughts, or mindfulness-based strategies aimed at acceptance and awareness? Several studies have compared the two treatments. In a large study in 2016 of patients with chronic low back pain, mindfulness and CBT were compared with the usual care, which was whatever care their primary care doctor provided them. The 342 participants were aged forty-nine, on average, and 80 percent reported having had back pain for at least a full year without a pain-free week. Mindfulness was as effective as CBT in improving symptoms of back pain as well as functional impairments, and participants in both groups also had similar improvements in catastrophizing and self-efficacy. Thus, at least for chronic low back pain, mindfulness appears to be as effective as commonly used CBT techniques.

In the study we completed in 2017, we evaluated whether CBT or a mindfulness-based approach is more effective for helping women deal with the distress associated with genital pain and which treatment leads to long-term retention of benefits. We were also interested in the characteristics of women who respond better to one treatment than the other so that clinicians will be able to make an informed decision about the best individualized treatment option.

Our findings mirrored those of several past studies: we found that women receiving CBT experienced significant declines in their genital pain and improvements in their distress, catastrophizing, pain hypervigilance, and sexual functioning. However, we also found that while women practicing mindfulness experience the same benefits as women receiving CBT, in the main outcome of women's self-reported pain during sexual activity, the women in the mindfulness group benefited even more than the women in the CBT group. The women's pain scores were reduced by over half in both groups, meaning that in addition to the well-accepted CBT approach, mindfulness-based therapy appears to be an equally suitable treatment option. Thus, the saying that tuning in trumps tuning out also appears to hold true for mindfulness-based treatment for genital pain.

These beneficial effects were maintained at six months and even at twelve months after women completed their work in groups. The participants reported that they appreciated learning a new way of experiencing their pain and that tuning in to the sensations of pain rather than distracting themselves from it, as they had done for years, offered a more effective way of managing their condition.

After participating in eight sessions of mindfulness-based therapy, and continuing with a daily meditation practice on her own, Sierra experienced a marked reduction in the distress associated with her chronic genital pain. She also reported that the pain during sex was far less than before she started meditating, and in some encounters she did not feel any genital pain at all. However, what was particularly meaningful for her was that her desire for sex returned. The more she focused on the sensations of Ali's hand touching her body, the less aversion she felt to his touch. Over time, she moved from aversion to neutrality to pleasure. She could focus on the warmth and comfort of his hand touching her body, and her worries about genital pain and any imagined catastrophic outcome were treated as background noise. She experienced firsthand the power of moving her attention to pleasurable sensations.

Within a few months, Sierra's sexual desire returned. This outcome was especially significant given that it challenged her belief that the loss of her desire meant that she and Ali lacked chemistry and were destined for separation. Although her sexual pain continued for the next few years, she learned to manage it through her practice of mindfulness, and the renewal of her sexual desire and arousal seemed to act as an analgesic for any residual vaginal pain. Sierra's case provides a powerful illustration of the brain → pain → sexual response → mindfulness cycle. Her story reminds us that, ultimately, a healthy sexual response resides in the brain—and that is exactly what mindfulness targets.

CHAPTER 10

YOU HAVE MY ATTENTION—
NOW WHAT?

The sense of touch is the special sense most used in sexual interchange.

MASTERS AND JOHNSON, Keynote Address,
"Sex Therapy on Its 25th Anniversary: Why It Survives"

INDFULNESS IS NOT a passing fad. It is not the latest late-night television gimmick guaranteed to change your life for only $39.99. Interest in it has sharply increased since the 1980s, with an exponential growth in the number of scientific publications evaluating it, and we do not predict that this interest will wane any time soon. The list of ailments, both medical and psychological, that have benefited from mindfulness is long and still growing. A Google search for "mindfulness" returns almost 78 million hits. By the time this book lands in your hands, that number is likely to have increased.

In addition to helping people with various clinical diagnoses, mindfulness has been used for specific symptoms. In August 2016, the *International Journal of Cardiology* published a study entitled "A randomized controlled trial evaluating mindfulness-based stress reduction (MBSR) for the treatment of palpitations: A pilot study," in which men and women with benign heart palpitations took part in mindfulness-based stress reduction. Those in the mindfulness group were found to have a significant decrease in the intensity of their heart palpitations, and these gains were maintained when the participants were tested a month after the program had ended. The researchers speculated that in addition to experiencing an overall reduction in the frequency of their heart palpitations, the participants worried less about those sensations when they were present, resulting in an overall decrease in the amount of psychological suffering while the heart was palpitating.

By studying the brain, we've learned much about how mindfulness translates into a variety of health-related improvements. The evidence points strongly to the conclusion that mindfulness ultimately changes the brain—its structure and its function. Mindfulness improves communication between different areas of the brain, allowing the individual to experience deeper states of consciousness. It is just as much "brain" as it is "mind" (though the term "mindfulness" is preferable to "brainfulness," as the latter may connote narcissism). Some argue that the distinction between the brain and the mind is artificial, especially since events of the mind are directly affected by, and in turn affect, activities of the brain.

Since the early days when Jon Kabat-Zinn taught mindfulness to a small group of patients with chronic and debilitating pain at the Center for Mindfulness at the University of Massachusetts, mindfulness has become a core component of childhood education and is used by the U.S. Department of Defense, Silicon Valley tech companies, massive corporations like General Mills and Google, leadership training programs, physician well-being training programs, and countless psychological clinics, institutes, and centers. When teaching participants across these vast populations, teachers often rely on discussing brain-related changes to communicate the power of mindfulness and invoke a curiosity about it.

This book has focused on mindfulness as a learned skill that can be used to cultivate sexual desire and to reduce genital discomfort. The exercises included here have been tested, critiqued, revised, tweaked, and tested again in hundreds of women, and we have published the findings from this program of research in several scientific journals (see brottolab. com and the references section of this book). We recorded our own mindfulness guides in a recording studio, in part so that the women listening to the recordings would hear a familiar voice and in part because we wanted to ensure that all parts of the body were mentioned during the Body Scan. In most (perhaps even all?) mindfulness guides provided online and in many mindfulness books, the Body Scan takes a leap from the belly to the hips to the thighs and lower legs, totally bypassing the genital area. In our recorded mindfulness guides, which we have provided to hundreds of women attending our groups, and in our training manuals, which thousands of people around the world have used, we deliberately invite women to pay attention to sensations in the abdomen, groin, pelvis, and vulva. We guide women to spend as much time focusing on sensations in their genitals as they spend paying attention to sensations in their neck and back and elsewhere. Although our long-term studies evaluating the mechanisms underlying how mindfulness cultivates sexual desire are still underway at the time of this writing, we believe that harnessing attention is key to sex-related success.

However, even if you have never practiced any of these mindfulness strategies, my bet is that you have tasted the power of mindfulness as it applies to sexuality already. Can you recall an instance in your life when you experienced a head-to-toe pleasing and satisfying sexual encounter? Maybe it was with your current partner? Maybe it was in your youth? Maybe it was during a time when you were feeling particularly experimental? Maybe it was on your own without a partner? Regardless of the details of the encounter, most people, including those who currently experience great difficulties with sexuality, can recall at least one such encounter when sex was simply sensational.

If you have experienced such an encounter, you can probably recall it with great vividness. You can probably recollect the location, the partner, the year, and many of the intimate details. Perhaps during this encounter you were not thinking about work or an exam or what you were going to do the next day. In fact, when people recollect their best sexual experiences, they describe a state of being fully present—fully alive and embodied. Over the last decade, psychologist Peggy Kleinplatz has been exploring what makes for optimal sex. She has interviewed countless men and women and posed the following question to them: What makes your sex great? Kleinplatz has received hundreds of responses to this question, including responses from a large number of sex therapists. In analyzing them, she and her team have identified eight main themes.

1. Respondents described being *completely present*, focused, embodied, and immersed.
2. Optimal sexual experiences involved a sense of connection and being *in sync*.
3. Deep intimacy accompanied *mutual respect and caring*.

4. *Communication was extraordinary*, both verbally and non-verbally.
5. Respondents viewed sex as an *adventure*.
6. They described sex as an opportunity to be *authentic, uninhib-ited, and totally free* with their partners.
7. They enjoyed the feeling of *vulnerability*.
8. Many described these optimal sexual experiences as *transformative*.

Couples interviewed who narrate experiences of optimal sexuality report in exquisite detail each sensation during an encounter. They often say that, in that moment, nothing else mattered or registered. In their recollections of wonderful sex, they were fully embodied, fully mindful. Perhaps it is no wonder that when people describe unpleasant sexual encounters, or unrewarding experiences, they also describe "wishing it were over" or bypassing the slow, deliberate touching characteristic of foreplay in favor of a quick progression straight to intercourse. People who have had optimal and transcendental sexual experiences also often discuss the quality of their interactions over the quantity of their interactions—a notion that runs counter to the much-touted "normalcy" of frequent, regular sex.

If you would like to begin a mindfulness program on your own or perhaps brush up on a practice that you had in the past, you might consider some of the common questions, concerns, and obstacles that women have posed to us before taking part in our groups.

Q. Do I need to meditate for hours every day in order to benefit from mindfulness?
A. Although many of the experts in mindfulness medita-tion emphasize the need for a structured daily meditation

practice, this does not mean that you need to quit your job to make room in your schedule to meditate. In the well-studied mindfulness-based stress reduction programs, participants engaged in approximately forty-five minutes of daily mindfulness practice over the course of their eight-week program, which also included a full-day retreat that consisted of silent walking and eating meditations. However, there is evidence that a shorter practice time might still be useful for cultivating awareness.

In one study published in 2007 that used integrative body-mind training, a combination of mindfulness meditation, relaxation, breathing exercises, and mental imagery, participants experienced a significant improvement in attention, anxiety, depression, anger, and fatigue compared with a control group after only five days of structured practice. Notably, these participants worked closely with a coach to help them refine their practice, and the researchers argued that this individualized feedback may have contributed to their speedy gains.

James Carmody and Ruth Baer, two mindfulness scientists from the United States, were interested in the question of whether the duration of a mindfulness program (in hours) was associated with improvements in psychological endpoints, such as anxiety, depression, and stress. They examined thirty studies that evaluated mindfulness-based stress reduction and found no association between the duration of the program and improvements in anxiety, depression, or stress. That said, most of the research evaluating mindfulness-based interventions has been based on programs that are eight weeks long or only slightly shorter.

Does the number of minutes one meditates each day affect the benefits one experiences from meditating? In a direct test of this, one study that recruited participants from six meditation centers around the Berkeley area compared the effects of minutes-per-day-of-meditation with the effects of the total number of hours spent meditating over one's lifetime. The researchers used the Stroop test, which, as you will recall, asks participants to name the color that the words "red," "green," or "blue" are printed in, meaning that participants must inhibit their natural tendency to read the words. The study found a significant association between the number of errors made and the number of minutes spent meditating per day. Those who meditated for more minutes per day made fewer errors. However, there was no association between the number of hours spent meditating over the course of one's lifetime and performance on the Stroop test.

Q. I am in a relationship with a man. Will mindfulness benefit my partner's sexuality in the same way it can boost my own?
A. The bulk of this book has focused on sexual desire, sexual motivation, and sexual pain in women, and we've considered in great detail the ways in which mindfulness may be useful. However, mindfulness has also been used effectively with men who experience sexual concerns, and I would predict that it affects mood, attention, distractions, bodily awareness, judgmental thoughts, and tuning in to genital sensations in a similar way as it is understood to affect women.

Mindfulness might be particularly helpful to men who experience situational difficulty with erections. This occurs when a man encounters no difficulties reaching or keeping an erection during solo sex play but has trouble getting or keeping an erection while having sex with a partner. In such situations, there may be no physiological cause, such as a

problem in the hardwiring of blood vessels and nerves sup-
plying the penis. One way of determining whether there are
physiological problems is to ask if the man is able to have
erections at night or immediately upon waking up—presum-
ably before psychological concerns, thoughts, or worries
set in.

If there is a physical cause, the man will have impaired
erections during the night and on waking, as well as in his
sexual encounters. If his erections seem normal at night or
in the early morning and are a problem only during sex, this
suggests (but does not guarantee, of course) a more psychological cause. Worries about the reliability of the erection,
thoughts about being a sexual failure, and concerns about
how his partner will respond if he loses his erection may elicit
enough anxiety to inhibit the erection. Moreover, the constant
worry that he won't get or be able to maintain an erection
means that the man is not paying attention to his bodily
sensations and connection with his partner in the present
moment and that, in turn, feedback from his genital response
is not reaching the brain.

In a study carried out in 1979, nine men with situational
erectile dysfunction were taught how to pay attention to their
genital sensations, such as tingling, and genital temperature
in their physician's office and then encouraged to practice
this twice daily thereafter. After two weeks of mindfulness
practice, those who did their homework were able to notice
and then increase the sensations of warmth in their penis and
had improved erections with sexual intercourse.

When assessed three months later, those men who were
successful at the two-week point continued to have good
erections with partnered sex. This study never quite triggered
a wave of interest among sex researchers and therapists,

however, and it is only recently that mindfulness has been once again tested in men with erectile difficulties. It may be that all the hoopla around Viagra and other oral medications for erectile problems overshadowed the psychological approaches and buried this research somewhere deep in the cobwebs of the Internet.

Mindfulness as a treatment for men with sexual concerns has recently been explored again. Dr. Jennifer Bossio, a postdoctoral fellow in my research laboratory at the University of British Columbia, collaborated with sexual medicine experts* in men's sexual functioning from the BC Centre for Sexual Medicine to investigate this topic. In this intervention, men with situational erectile difficulties took part in four group sessions lasting two hours each. For half of each session, the men participated in many of the same meditations outlined earlier in this book for women, and for the other half they learned about the inhibitors and facilitators of erections and of men's sexual response more generally.

As the men considered the impact of their distractions and preoccupations on their ability to have erections, those who were using Viagra (and similar medications) but not finding them to be consistently helpful discovered that when they are distracted and not paying attention to sexual cues, these medications will not work. They also began to understand how mindfulness could be used to increase their focus on erotic triggers and so boost the efficacy of the medications they were using.

The men were unanimous in finding the sessions useful. They noted that they were highly skeptical at the beginning

---

* *These sexual medicine experts in men's sexual functioning were Rosemary Basson, Shauna Correia, Stacy Elliott, and Miriam Driscoll.*

about the extent to which "attention manipulation" would help
with their erections, but they committed to the practice any-
way (likely because conventional oral medications were not
as effective for them as they had hoped). They quickly over-
came any hesitations they had about speaking about their
sexual concerns with other men. They dove head first into the
material and into the daily meditation practices. One participant told us:

> I think the sessions were helpful in reducing the distraction.
> And the distraction being these worrying thoughts, anxious
> thoughts. So for me, I'm just trying to go back and visualize
> myself focusing on the moment, I guess, and as a result of
> that, I guess reducing the anxious or worrying thoughts that
> happen during sex.

Although this study was small, it provides promise for
sex therapists, sex researchers, and others keen to explore
mindfulness-based approaches with men who have sexual
difficulties. We hope that a book for men similar to this one
appears in the near future.

Q. I am an atheist. Can I still meditate?
A. I have observed that each time a story about mindfulness
is covered in our community newspaper, at least a few people
write in to the paper to protest what they see as a religious
practice being promoted in schools. Such reactions reflect a
misunderstanding about mindfulness-based interventions as
taught in our secular Western culture and in our schools, community centers, clinics, and hospitals.

Mindfulness has a long history in the West, accompanied by a parallel scientifically motivated effort to test the

evidence-based aspects of mindfulness on health and well-being. But it has a much, much longer history in the East, where mindfulness has been a core aspect of Buddhist teaching and is described in the Buddhist text the *Satipatthana Sutta*. This text provides a series of practices that allow the practitioner to develop the mental quality of mindfulness, which reflects attention, alertness, and an equanimity toward all sensations, thoughts, and feelings that arise.

Although mindfulness as taught in mindfulness-based therapy shares many similarities with mindful observation in Buddhism, the two approaches differ in important ways. Both cultivate concentration through focusing on a target and guiding the mind back to the target as it wanders. And both also may lead to the development of insight, which is defined as a firsthand experiential understanding of the present moment by knowing that sensations are not permanent. (Part of the development of insight is also understanding that there is not a "self" that exists separately from these experiences, and through repeated practice, one learns that sensations arise and fade somewhat independently from an individual "self" experiencing them.) However, mindfulness-based interventions differ from mindfulness practice in Buddhist teaching in that the former does not specifically train ethical behavior, which Buddhist scripts outline as the social rules of proper behavior. Also, within Buddhist traditions, mindfulness is situated within a framework that is oriented toward nonharming, or examining how meditative practices calm the mind and therefore relieve human suffering. A third way in which secular mindfulness and Buddhist mindfulness differ is that within the former, there may be little consideration for how the practices may trigger profound insights, whereas these are identified and worked with in the latter.

One of our team members, Dr. Andrea Grabovac, a psychiatrist, mindfulness teacher, writer, and clinician in Vancouver, together with her colleagues developed the Buddhist Psychological Model, which summarizes the underlying teaching of Buddhist texts and provides a simpler interpretation than that described in classic Buddhist texts of how mindfulness improves clinical well-being. When viewed through this lens, the essential elements of mindfulness practice, stripped of their religious undertones, become evident. As Grabovac, Mark Lau, and Brandilyn Willett, mental health–care providers and meditation teachers in Vancouver, note in their 2011 paper, mindfulness practice has three essential elements: alertness, receptivity, and equanimity. Rather than reacting habitually to thoughts as we normally do, being alert to sensations as they arise (whether they are physical or mental sensations) allows one to act more reflectively than reflexively. Receptivity is the practice of being open to any and all sensations—whether positive, negative, or neutral—and adopting a stance of "welcoming all the guests." When you are receptive, you may move your attention from object to object, or thought to thought, without trying to suppress your attention. Equanimity is the aspect of mindfulness that treats all arising experiences and emotions equally—the good, the bad, and the ugly. Modern-day practitioners of mindfulness emphasize that it is available, accessible, and useful regardless of any religious affiliation or lack thereof. It does not teach religion or require it.

Mindfulness practice, as described in this book and as taught in other mindfulness interventions like mindfulness-based stress reduction (MBSR), is not affiliated with Buddhism and does not rely on an understanding of Buddhist teaching in order for one to practice, learn from, and benefit from it. In fact, Jon Kabat-Zinn, when introducing mindfulness to Western medicine in the late 1970s through his work with sufferers of chronic pain, deliberately decontextualized mindfulness from its association with rows of monks in Lotus pose, and transformed it into an accessible practice that anyone could adopt. Throughout his teaching and writing, Kabat-Zinn emphasizes the universality of mindfulness: it is an inherent *human* capacity. So, welcome, Christians, Jews, Hindus, Sikhs, Muslims, people of all religious affiliations, atheists, and agnostics. Mindfulness is yours to practice.

Q. My mind wanders constantly. I just can't "do" mindfulness.
A. During our mindfulness exercises at the University of British Columbia, we engage in a thirty-to-forty-minute mindfulness exercise as a group during each of the eight sessions. After the formal "practice" is over, one of the group facilitators leads an inquiry, during which she will ask members of the group what they noticed during their mindfulness meditation. We have considered some of the components of the three-question inquiry in early chapters already, as it is an opportunity for the group participants themselves to ponder how paying attention to the raisin/breath/body sensations/sounds/thoughts of the mind may be relevant to their sexual concerns. Some women comment on specific sensations in their body. Others comment on the process of guiding their mind toward a certain target. Many state that they observed aspects of the present moment that they typically do not pay attention to. However, we also often hear something along the lines of "I cannot do this. I'm not wired that way."

In a recent group I co-led with a junior therapist, after our meditation on the raisin I asked the group what sensations they noticed during our practice. Jane was the first to speak up: "I found it boring. In the same way that I found yoga boring and so stopped. My brain is just not wired in that way. I'm not able to focus on one task. I'm a multitasker by nature." Jane may have been explaining why she found the instructions to focus on and observe the raisin to be challenging. However, she may also have been declaring at the outset that she simply did not want to practice mindfulness, despite all that it promised.

As a group facilitator, I have been faced with this challenging situation many times. How do I convey the promise of what mindfulness offers without appearing to be a salesperson? How do I respect where the person is while at the same time offering a glimpse of the wonderful gift that mindfulness offers if one just takes a chance and plunges in, leaving judgment and negative expectations behind? And how do I shield the other group members from the possible negative effects of this message?

Influenced by my own teachers, I respond by validating the experiences of women like Jane. I might say the following:

Jane, your experience is so common. So normal. Multitasking and mind wandering come about so automatically, and for many of us, it can feel like this is our natural state of being. Something that we cannot change, and something that is not worth changing. However, it is not our natural way of being. Consider a child playing in a field of flowers. That child focuses intently and intensely on every individual petal of the dandelion before her. She blows and watches with amazement as each one flakes off the stem and dances in the sky above her, swaying back and forth. That child is not worried about where the petal will land but is caught up in the moment of being with that petal as it floats through the air. With age, life experiences, and stress, our natural ability to be in the moment becomes suppressed as we face the onslaught of ever-present demands in our life. We come to believe that focusing on one thing at a time will prevent us from accomplishing anything at all. We stomp through the field of dandelions and don't even notice them anymore.

Many women can relate to this description of mindfulness as something that is inherently part of all of us but that has had to be suppressed to make room for the "doing" of life. We must remember that mindfulness is not about mastering the ability to fixate on a single object for hours on end, with a focused and sustained attention; it is about noticing when we are judging ourselves. When we catch ourselves thinking "This won't work" and see that as a mental event, we have already brought ourselves back to the present.

NOT ABOUT FIXING WHAT IS BROKEN

PEOPLE SEEK THERAPY for sexual difficulties because they want their issues to be resolved. They recall a time in their life that was free of sexual complaints, perhaps a time when concerns about their relationship did not affect that relationship or prospects of a relationship. Understandably, their distress leads them to identify a provider with expertise in fixing sexual problems, and for most people, this "reaching out" takes immense courage. Because sexuality is such a sensitive topic, people tend to suffer in silence. Unlike pharmacological treatments, however—and arguably most nonmindfulness-based psychological interventions—mindfulness does not aim to change anything. Mindfulness is ultimately about observing what is present and identifying thoughts about wanting an experience to be more than simply "passing mental events." A mindfulness-based approach to sexual dysfunction involves encouraging an individual to tune in to their current experience.

How does this tuning in resolve suffering? Thomas Borkovec, a retired psychology professor from Pennsylvania State University, describes it succinctly in his 2002 paper "Life in the Future Versus Life in the Present," as follows:

> If a focus on the outcome and the extrinsic aspects of an activity are conducive to anxiety and depression, then the objective quality of my work, whether washing dishes or writing grant proposals, will likely be lowered, given what we know about the adverse effects of negative emotion on performance. So seeking the extrinsic outcome makes the failure to achieve that outcome more likely. A focus on the process and intrinsic qualities of an activity reduces the likelihood of anxiety and depression (thus eliminating their negative impact on performance), increases the pleasure of joy during the process, and thus increases the likelihood of achieving the extrinsic outcome. I have to let go of the desired outcome in order to acquire it. What a paradoxical and strange way to live.

If we relate this directly to sexual concerns, focusing on imagined disastrous outcomes (for example, "My sexual response is dwindling and my partner will leave me") contributes to the likelihood of having a low-level sexual response. A mindful solution to this situation is to focus on the present moment—the sensations during sexual activity, both in the body and on the mind. Once you let go of the desire to change, the pathway toward achieving that change is less obscure. The most efficient path from A to B, through a mindfulness lens, is to have your feet firmly planted right at A.

CHAPTER 11

THE NEXT CHAPTER
OF THE PRESENT MOMENT

The real meditation is how you live your life.

JON KABAT-ZINN at Thrive, the Huffington Post's
second Third Metric conference

I F YOU ARE inspired by the exercises outlined in this book, you may wish to learn, practice, and incorporate sensate focus in its advanced stages into your life as a next step. Or you may find yourself avoiding activities such as sensate focus or any of the other mindfulness exercises described here. This is common, and you are not alone. Avoidance features front and center with sexual difficulties. As noted earlier, women who experience low sexual desire avoid potential sexual situations, such as undressing in front of a partner, kissing, and even going to bed at the same time. The avoidance is a Band-Aid that shields one from anticipated anxiety or disappointment during a sexual encounter. Over time, however, avoidance fuels anxiety and leads to more disappointment. The more you avoid these potentially sexual cues and situations, the more intense the anxiety becomes. Before you know it, the avoidance, which served a useful purpose at one point (because it kept anxiety and disappointment at bay), is now directly contributing to the sexual concerns themselves.

Take thirty-four-year-old Anita, for example. Avoidance has become the primary culprit behind her sexual difficulties. Despite being bombarded with sexual images and messages throughout her adult life, Anita's sexual experiences were unrewarding, awkward, and even painful. When she first became sexually active, at age eighteen, she believed that the pain she experienced during intercourse with her boyfriend was normal. An aunt had once told her that the first time she had intercourse her hymen would be ruptured and she would bleed, and at first she attributed her vaginal pain to this "normal event."

However, now in her mid-thirties and in a three-year relationship, although her sexual encounters are still somewhat painful, Anita's avoidance of all forms of intimacy has become her more significant sexual concern. In fact, she increasingly finds herself avoiding sex by going to sleep earlier than her partner, undressing only behind a locked door, and moving away when her partner starts to give her a kiss. It is not that Anita dislikes physical intimacy or connection with her partner, but she has come to avoid any activity that might lead to her partner becoming aroused and thus wanting sex. She is anxious for days leading up to vacations, when she is expected to be more sexual. She has even faked an illness to avoid going away on vacation with her partner. At the same time, she worries that her partner will leave her for someone who is more sexual.

Can paying attention help disrupt the pattern of avoidance? How might tuning in lead her to break free from the stickiness of avoidance?

Mindfulness offers a solution. By learning to observe her anxiety (anxious thoughts, feelings, behaviors, and sensations), Anita could start to no longer fear it. Her mindfulness practices allowed her to label avoidance as something to observe. She began to pay attention to and label the sensations in her body as she was drawn to avoidance. She observed that her avoidance had become a learned response to an anticipated dangerous situation. With repeated practice focusing on the sensations associated with avoidance, she began to no longer fear it. She viewed avoidance as a "guest" at the door. When she began to practice mindfulness with a partner present, the anxiety typically triggered by a partner began to lessen.

Other women and their partners, like Anita, discover that with time, if the couple can touch one another during a mindful practice, the touch itself, and the sensations emerging from the points of contact, can become a focus of present-moment awareness. Even when the tendency toward avoidance is present, they can observe those sensations along with other positive and desired sensations at the same time. The sky then becomes the limit for the kinds of touches that are exchanged while the woman and her partner breathe together and experience together, mindfully.

All of the skills practiced in mindful awareness—noticing bodily sensations, being aware of the breath, observing sounds and thoughts—can be directly applied to sexual activity with a partner. By now, you may have taken the plunge and attempted the various exercises outlined in this book. You can bring the same skills in present-moment, nonjudgmental, focused attention to your experiences with sexual activity. Moreover, because you may be experiencing some degree of sexual arousal, practicing mindfulness can be a wonderful opportunity to observe and *move in even closer* to the sensations that unfold during sexual arousal. This can take you a step closer to Peggy Kleinplatz's notion of optimal sex that perhaps at an earlier time seemed unreachable. Now it may be within your grasp, or perhaps just out of reach because of where your mind is. Your mind, which may have been your greatest foe in your quest to experience sexual satisfaction, may now become your greatest ally.

THE QUESTIONS THAT REMAIN

DESPITE ALL OF the advances in applying mindfulness to women's sexuality and the countless women who as a result of mindfulness have regained sexual feelings that they had lost for years, many questions remain. For example, how precisely does mindfulness work to improve sexual functioning in women? How exactly does paying attention to the intricacies of the breath translate into feelings of sexual desire? How long do the benefits of mindfulness persist after women stop participating in a mindfulness program, and how much ongoing daily practice is necessary to maintain these gains? Can mindfulness improve orgasm frequency and quality? Can mindfulness reverse the effects of aging and menopause on sexual functioning? And how does mindfulness compare with medication in cultivating women's sexual desire? Although we have no clear answers to any of these questions at time of writing, researchers around the world who have become intrigued with the power of mindful sex are beginning to explore them.

If we were to compare mindfulness with the pharmacological treatments available, other psychological interventions, and the mile-high list of aids and inducers that can be found in your local adult-only retail store or in the pages of *Cosmopolitan* magazine, I believe that we would find it the most effective antidote against sexual dysfunction. I may be criticized for holding this view without the mass of research that is needed before such conclusions can be reached (although there is never "proof" of a theory, but rather an accumulation of strong evidence that no effect—the null hypothesis—is unlikely). However, we do have enough evidence of the transformative effects of mindfulness on sexuality, and in many other aspects of health and well-being associated with sexuality, that I feel comfortable defending my position tenaciously.

THE MOST IMPORTANT INGREDIENT IN SATISFYING SEX

AS OF 2017, a growing body of research has shown mindfulness to be important for sexual functioning and sexual satisfaction. Based on my own observation of mindfulness, I would argue that satisfying sex is quite simply *not possible* without mindfulness. When the women in our groups recall an experience of magnificent sex, the details of the activities and settings vary significantly. However, their stories share one critical ingredient in common: the person was *fully present*. Fully alive. Fully connected. Fully there. Acrobatic sex or willful stamina are not what make sex truly magnificent. In my opinion, it is mindfulness. To be fully present with each sensation, without judgment or commentary, is what I think has been missing from sex for the countless women who are dissatisfied with sex. It cannot be packaged up in a little pink pill. It cannot be injected or placed on the arm in patch form. It is simple but not easy. It requires a lifetime commitment to practice.

Mindfulness is transformational. I invite you to begin to experience sex in a way you never have before. It is all within reach, simply by paying attention. Right now. Right where you are.

WHERE TO FIND HELP

I T MAY NOT be difficult to locate a mindfulness teacher in most large cities. In smaller communities, I encourage you to contact your local community center to see if it offers the eight-week mindfulness-based stress reduction (MBSR) program or mindfulness-based cognitive therapy (MBCT). Such programs are typically delivered to groups of six to fifteen individuals, whether women-only or mixed sex, and provides an atmosphere of support and camaraderie. For those who prefer to learn mindfulness individually, clinicians, therapists, and teachers who are experienced in mindful meditation, or who are certified mindfulness practitioners, are also spread throughout North America. The Center for Mindfulness in Boston at the University of Massachusetts Medical School, where Jon Kabat-Zinn's foundational work in developing the eight-week mindfulness program started, also provides an excellent resource for locating mindfulness programs, retreats, and intensive workshops across North America. The center also offers an eight-week mindfulness program entirely online.

There are also a variety of apps for smartphones that are designed to provide guidance in mindfulness practice. One favorite of mine is Headspace, developed by Andy Puddicombe, a former Tibetan Buddhist monk who left university to travel to Nepal, India, Burma, Thailand, Australia, and Russia. When he returned to London, he turned his attention to making mindfulness accessible to the masses. After years of development, he launched Headspace in 2010. The app houses myriad recorded mindfulness guides of varying duration. It can be customized to suit the listener's interests, such as mindfulness to cope with distractions, anxiety, or pain. It also provides an opportunity to track your practice. I often suggest to those who are interested in getting a taste of mindfulness to try the Headspace app for a month.

Are there clinicians who specialize in sexuality and treating sexual problems that have experience and expertise in teaching mindfulness? Yes, there are. However, they may be difficult to find, since there is no central online repository of mindfulness and sexuality experts, and so if you are interested in locating such an expert, it may take a bit of effort. There are directories of sex therapists, such as the following:

- American Association of Sexuality Educators, Counselors and Therapists (aasect.org), which allows you to locate a sexuality counselor who is a member of AASECT in a number of different countries.
- The Society for Sex Therapy and Research (sstarnet.org) offers a similar resource to identify sex therapists who are also SSTAR members, mostly in North America.
- Ontario is the only Canadian province with a directory of sex therapists: the Board of Examiners in Sex Therapy and Counselling in Ontario (bestco.info).

Unfortunately, these directories do not indicate whether the professional has experience in teaching clients mindfulness. However, a quick perusal of their website or a brief telephone call can provide this information.

SELECT BIBLIOGRAPHY

American Psychological Association (2017). *Stress in America: Coping with change* [Press release]. Released February 15, 2017. Retrieved from apa. org/news/press/releases/stress/index.aspx

Angel, K. (2010). The history of "female sexual dysfunction" as a mental disorder in the 20th century. *Current Opinions in Psychiatry, 23*, 536-541.

Arnow, B. A., Millheiser, L., Garrett, A., Polan, M. L., Glover, G. H., Hill, K. R., ... & Buchanan, T. (2009). Women with hypoactive sexual desire disorder compared to normal females: A functional magnetic resonance imaging study. *Neuroscience, 158*(2), 484-502.

Atlantis, E., & Sullivan, T. (2012). Bidirectional association between depression and sexual dysfunction: A systematic review and meta-analysis. *Journal of Sexual Medicine, 9*, 1497-1507.

Basson, R. (2000). The female sexual response: A different model. *Journal of Sex & Marital Therapy, 26*(1), 51-65.

Borkovec, T. D. (2002). Life in the future versus life in the present. *Clinical Psychology: Science and Practice, 9*(1), 76-80.

Brotto, L. A. (2010). The DSM diagnostic criteria for hypoactive sexual desire disorder in women. *Archives of Sexual Behavior, 39*, 221-239.

Brotto, L. A., & Basson, R. (2014). Group mindfulness-based therapy significantly improves sexual desire in women. *Behaviour Research and Therapy, 57*, 43-54.

Brotto, L. A., Erskine, Y., Carey, M., Ehlen, T., Finlayson, S., Heywood, M., ...
& Miller, D. (2012). A brief mindfulness-based cognitive behavioral
intervention improves sexual functioning versus wait-list control
in women treated for gynecologic cancer. *Gynecologic Oncology*, 125(2),
320-325.

Brotto, L. A., Seal, B. N., & Rellini, A. (2012). Pilot study of a brief cognitive
behavioral versus mindfulness-based intervention for women with
sexual distress and a history of childhood sexual abuse. *Journal of Sex &
Marital Therapy*, 38(1), 1-27.

Carmody, J., & Baer, R. A. (2009). How long does a mindfulness-based
stress reduction program need to be? A review of class contact hours
and effect sizes for psychological distress. *Journal of Clinical Psychology*,
65(6), 627-638.

Cryle, P. (2009). "A terrible ordeal from every point of view": (Not) managing female sexuality on the wedding night. *Journal of the History of
Sexuality*, 18(1), 44-64.

Cyranowski, J. M., Bromberger, J., Youk, A., Matthews, K., Kravitz, H. M.,
& Powell, L. H. (2004). Lifetime depression history and sexual function in women at midlife. *Archives of Sexual Behavior*, 33(6), 539-548.

Dennerstein, L., Guthrie, J. R., Hayes, R. D., DeRogatis, L. R., & Lehert, P.
(2008). Sexual function, dysfunction, and sexual distress in a prospective, population-based sample of mid-aged, Australian-born women.
The Journal of Sexual Medicine, 5(10), 2291-2299.

Farb, N. A., Segal, Z. V., Mayberg, H., Bean, J., McKeon, D., Fatima, Z., &
Anderson, A. K. (2007). Attending to the present: Mindfulness meditation reveals distinct neural modes of self-reference. *Social Cognitive
and Affective Neuroscience*, 2(4), 313-322.

Frühauf, S., Gerger, H., Schmidt, H. M., Munder, T., & Barth, J. (2013).
Efficacy of psychological interventions for sexual dysfunction: A
systematic review and meta-analysis. *Archives of Sexual Behavior*, 42(6),
915-933.

Grabovac, A. D., Lau, M. A., & Willett, B. R. (2011). Mechanisms of mindfulness: A Buddhist psychological model. *Mindfulness, 2*(3), 154-166.

Hanh, T. N. (2016). *The miracle of mindfulness*. Boston: Beacon Press.

Harding, K. (2015). *Asking for it: The alarming rise of rape culture—and what we can do about it*. Boston: Da Capo Lifelong Books.

Kabat-Zinn, J. (1990). *Full catastrophe living: Using the wisdom of your body and mind to face stress, pain, and illness*. New York: Delacorte Press.

Kleinplatz, P. J., Ménard, A. D., Paquet, M. P., Paradis, N., Campbell, M., Zuccarino, D., & Mehak, L. (2009). The components of optimal sexuality: A portrait of "great sex." *The Canadian Journal of Human Sexuality, 18*(1-2), 1-13.

Kocsis, A., & Newbury-Helps, J. (2016). Mindfulness in sex therapy and intimate relationships (MSIR): Clinical protocol and theory development. *Mindfulness, 7*(3), 690-699.

Laumann, E. O., Paik, A., & Rosen, R. C. (1999). Sexual dysfunction in the United States: Prevalence and predictors. *Journal of the American Medical Association, 281*(6), 537-544.

Masters, W. H., & Johnson, V. E. (1970). *Human sexual inadequacy*. Boston: Little, Brown.

Meston, C. M., & Buss, D. M. (2007). Why humans have sex. *Archives of Sexual Behavior, 36*(4), 477-507.

Mitchell, K. R., Mercer, C. H., Ploubidis, G. B., Jones, K. G., Datta, J., Field, N., ... & Clifton, S. (2013). Sexual function in Britain: Findings from the third National Survey of Sexual Attitudes and Lifestyles (Natsal-3). *The Lancet, 382*(9907), 1817-1829.

Paterson, L. Q., Handy, A. B., & Brotto, L. A. (2016). A pilot study of eight-session mindfulness-based cognitive therapy adapted for women's sexual interest/arousal disorder. *The Journal of Sex Research, 54*(7), 850-861.

Perelman, M. A. (2014). The history of sexual medicine. In D. L. Tolman & L. M. Diamond (eds.), *APA handbook of sexuality and psychology: Volume 2:*

Contextual Approaches (pp. 137-179).Washington: American Psychological Association.

Pickert, K. (February 3, 2014). The mindful revolution. *Time*, pp. 34-48.

Shifren, J. L., Monz, B. U., Russo, P. A., Segreti, A., & Johannes, C. B. (2008). Sexual problems and distress in United States women: Prevalence and correlates. *Obstetrics & Gynecology*, 112(5), 970-978.

Tiefer, L. (1991). Historical, scientific, clinical and feminist criticisms of "the human sexual response cycle" model. *Annual Review of Sex Research*, 2(1), 1-23.

Weiner, L., & Avery-Clark, C. (2017). *Sensate focus in sex therapy: The illustrated manual*. New York: Routledge.

Wilson, G. (2005). The "infomania" study. Accessed at news.bbc.co.uk/2/hi/uk_news/4471607.stm

ACKNOWLEDGMENTS

MY PERSONAL AND professional journey in mindfulness began at a pivotal time of transition in my life while at the University of Washington, Seattle, USA. I am indebted to Dr. Amy Wagner and Dr. Craig Sawchuk, my residency supervisors there, for introducing me to mindfulness and for providing me with the nudge I needed to explore this practice with women experiencing sexual concerns. I am grateful to Dr. Julia Heiman, my former postdoctoral fellowship supervisor and ongoing mentor, who not only worked with me tirelessly in exploring how mindfulness might be incorporated into the lives of cancer survivors who had lost their sense of sexual arousal but also co-wrote the first treatment manual with me. To Dr. Rosemary Basson, for your gentle presence, your cogent articulation of women's sexual response, and your unwavering support and collaboration as this work in mindfulness-based approaches for women evolved over the past decade, I am forever grateful to you. In addition to being my mentor, teacher, and advocate, you have also been a tremendous friend.

Thank you to the many mindfulness teachers who influenced this work, including Dr. Andrea Grabovac and Dr. Mark

Lau, and to Dr. Jon Kabat-Zinn, who engaged in a dialogue about how the Body Scan might be adapted for women with sexual and body concerns.

The team of clinicians and scientists who contributed to the evolution of our treatment manuals is long, but I particularly wish to acknowledge and thank Marie Carlson, Dr. Miriam Driscoll, Dr. Mijal Luria, Dr. Laurel Paterson, Monique Rees, and Dr. Kelly Smith for the endless hours of discussion, adaptation, testing, revising, refining, and re-testing of the exercises. Thank you to the amazing team of dedicated students and research staff at the University of British Columbia Sexual Health Laboratory, who worked hard to ensure our mindfulness groups were full, women's questions were answered, and our data collection was complete. Each of you teaches me more than I can deliver in return, and I thank you for making our lab a family. To my community of sex researchers and clinicians who provided thoughtful questions and critiques every time I presented our findings at scientific meetings, each of your comments have shaped this work over time, and I feel grateful to belong to such a small but smart group of sex therapists and researchers. In particular, I wish to thank my friend and collaborator, Dr. Meredith Chivers, whose work and passion for improving the science of women's experiences significantly shapes my own. I'd also like to express a grateful thank you to Dr. David Goldmeier, my kindred spirit in this journey.

To the team at Greystone Books, and in particular, my editor, Nancy Flight, who patiently nudged me from 2009 to 2015 to consider writing this book. Nancy, your steadfast support and honest feedback throughout this writing has been greatly appreciated. Thank you for convincing me that scientists can learn to write for the masses. Thank you to owner and publisher, Rob Sanders, who showed enthusiasm for the topic even when it felt like a foreign language! Alice Fleerackers and the marketing team, and Lesley Cameron, the superb editorial consultant who provided an attention to detail that mindfulness can only envy, your assistance was invaluable.

As for my family, I want to thank Danica, Sebastian, and Luca for demonstrating the simplicity of mindfulness through the eyes of a child. Thank you also for never questioning the endless hours that is required of a clinician-scientist-writer. I hope the words in this book guide each of your own lives and that you discover what truly makes you happy in love and life. To my husband, Ed Fontana, who has journeyed with me throughout the evolution of mindful sex and participated enthusiastically at every stage, I love you. Rentato and Germana Brotto, my parents, the values you instilled in me of perseverance and the pursuit of excellence guide everything I do personally and professionally. I will never forget the humble roots we came from. To the many incredible friends who have shared in dialogue about sex and happiness over the twenty years of my career, your stories, support, laughter, and honesty are woven throughout this book. You are my community of sisters. This includes my academic sisters who share the same experiences, making explanations unnecessary, including Dr. Robin Milhausen, Dr. Lucia O'Sullivan, and Dr. Elke Reissing.

Finally, a book about mindfulness for women would simply not be possible without the countless women who have participated in our groups. Thank you to those women and to the many clients I have been privileged to work with individually and as couples. Your healthy skepticism about how tuning in can trump tuning out kept me straight on the path of discovery, and I hope that the evidence you helped to generate can be useful to each of you personally. I carry each of your stories with me, the stories of grief and frustration, the stories of loss and aging, and the stories of ecstasy and new discovery with an old partner. Thank you for trusting that the space we shared to cultivate this gift of nonjudgmental awareness was sacred and private. This book is dedicated to you and your relationships.

INDEX